End of Covid-19 (Corona Virus)Intection

Vol-II

Covid-19 Virus infection will be over on 27th June 2022

(Indian Astrology based prediction)

Pradeep Saxena

This book is written to pacify the people from the chaos due to the wide spread typical virus of the century-"Corona-Covid-19 Virus" , spreading throughout the world on the basis of Indian Astrology.

The analysis is as accurate and reliable as possible .

Both the publisher and the author of this book are in no way expert on the topics discussed in this book. The whole analysis is made herein only for entertainment purpose.

No part of this book can be challenged in any court of law.

No part of this book may be quoted from or reproduced in any form by means such as printing, scanning, photocopying, or otherwise without prior written permission of the copyright holder.

There are no scenarios in which the publisher or the original author of this book can be in any way deemed liable for any hardship or damages that may befall them after understanding information described herein

Dedicated

To

My Daughters

Alpna & Aditi

Contents

Introduction

The first case of Corona Virus (Covid-19) was detected in Wuhan province of China on 10th December 2019, the first death due to Covid-19 virus took place in China on 11th January 2020.Since then hundreds of millions of people have been infecting by this virus. Millions of people have died due to this virus.

For the last one year huge chaos is there among people throughout the world. To overcome the fear of Covid-19 virus, I have tried to let the people know when Covid-19 virus infection rate will increase or decrease so that they may take precautions accordingly.

I have tried to analyze spreading of Covid-19 virus on the basis of Indian Astrology.

I found that on 16th November 2019, when Covid-19 was discovered (as per Guardian news paper), Soft planets (as per Indian Astrology) –Moon, Mercury, Venus and Jupiter were under the effects of Rough planets (as per Indian Astrology)-Sun, Marsh, Saturn, Rahu and Ketu. On 11th January 2020 (the day when first death took place due to Covid-19 virus), again all the four soft planets were under the effects of all the five rough planets.

From this it can be concluded that when any of the four soft planets will go on under the effects of any of the five rough planets, Covid-19 infection/deaths will go on continuing .The effect of Covid-19 virus will be over only when this chain of effects of soft planets by rough planets be broken.

By analyzing the daily motions of all the nine planets, it is concluded that on 27th June 2022, for the first time all the four soft planets will come out from the effects of rough planets. Hence as per my astrological analysis , Covid-19 virus infection will be over on 27th June 2022.

At the beginning of this book , I have explained some basic concepts of Indian Astrology in easy steps so that who are not familiar with Indian Astrology may also understand this book easily without taking assistance of any other book or person.

Chapter 1

Evolution of Covid-19 Virus

If the facts shown by China be believed ,then very first a 57 years lady Mrs. V. Guiksan from Sea Food Market of Wuhan province of China was infected from Covid-19 virus on 10th Dec. 2019.However the govt. of Wuhan province said that first of all a Mr. Chin was infected from Covid-19 virus and also said, he never visited the sea food market. But Wuhan govt. did not disclosed when Mr. Chin was infected.

On the other hand, as per the Guardian newspaper ,the first case of infection of Covid-19 came on 16th November 2019.

The first death due to Covid-19 virus took place on 11th jan.2019 in Wuhan province.

As per Indian Astrology, the planet Jupiter entered into Sagittarius zodiac group on 4th November 2019.

Planetary position on 4th November 2019 (As per Indian Astrology)----

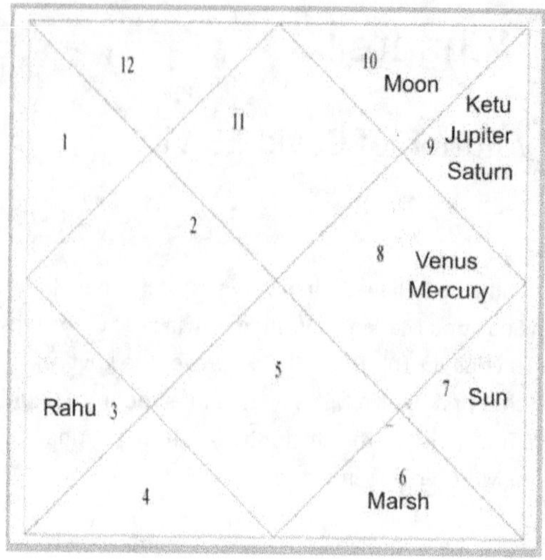

As soon as the planet Jupiter entered into the Sagittarius zodiac group, it came under the effect of Saturn, Rahu and ketu. Further the fourth fullsight of Marsh from Virgo zodiac group was also on Jupiter. By 6th November 2019,Mercury and Venus were moving in Scorpio zodiac group. No effect of rough planets –Sun, Marsh, Saturn, Rahu or ketu were on these planets.

On 7th November 2019,the planet Mercury entered into Libra zodiac group with retarding motion. Now it came under the effect of Sun, further fifth full sight of Rahu was also on Mercury.

On 10th November 2019,the planet Marsh entered into Libra zodiac group. Now the planet Mercury came into the effect of rough planets Sun and Marsh along with fifth full sight of Rahu. Full seventh sights of Sun and Marsh were also on Moon (moving in Aries zodiac group).

The planets Moon, Venus, Mercury and Jupiter are known as Soft planets and Rahu, ketu, Sun, Marsh and Saturn are known as rough or hard planets in Indian astrology.

On 17th November 2019,the planet Sun moved into the zodiac group Scorpio

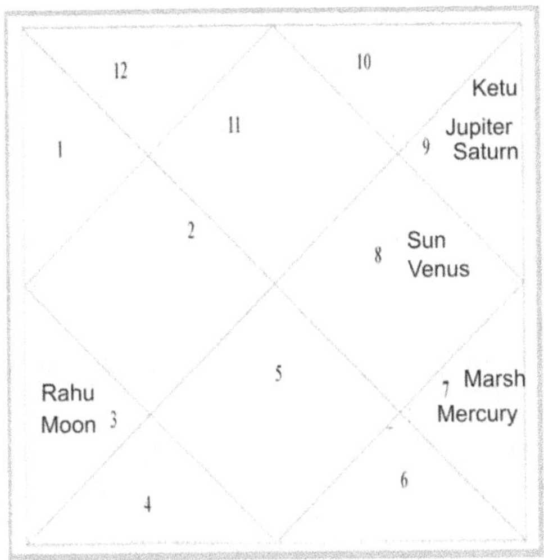

<u>Planetary position on 17th November 2019 (As per Indian Astrology)--</u>

Now the planet Moon was under the effect of Rahu, Ketu and Saturn. Mercury was under the effects of Marsh and Rahu (Full fifth sight of Rahu),Venus was under the effect of Sun, and Jupiter was under the effects of Rahu (Seventh full sight), Ketu, Saturn .

Hence on 17th November 2019, all the four soft planets Moon, Jupiter, Venus and Mercury came under the effects of rough planets Rahu, ketu, Saturn, Sun and Marsh. From this It can be concluded that Covid-19 virus came to effect on 17th November 2019 in Vuhan province of China

_The first death due to Covid-19 virus in China took place on 11th Jan.2020.

<u>Planetary position on 11th jan.2020 (As per Indian Astrology)</u>----

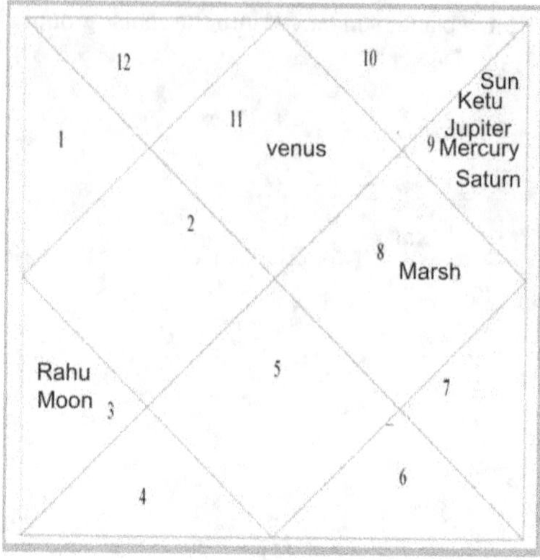

On 11th Jan. 2020,soft planets Mercury and Jupiter were under the effects of Sun, Saturn, Rahu and Ketu .The planet Venus was under the effects of Marsh and Rahu while Moon was under the effects of Rahu, ketu, Sun and Saturn.

From these it can be concluded that when the soft planets moon, Jupiter, Mercury and Venus be not under the effects of any of the rough planets Sun, Saturn, Marsh ,Rahu or Ketu,the Covid-19 virus effect will be over.

Chapter 2

Some basic concepts of Indian Astrology

To make the explanation easy ,we should know some basic

Concepts of Indian Astrology

Positions of Various houses in a Horoscope –(Chart-1)

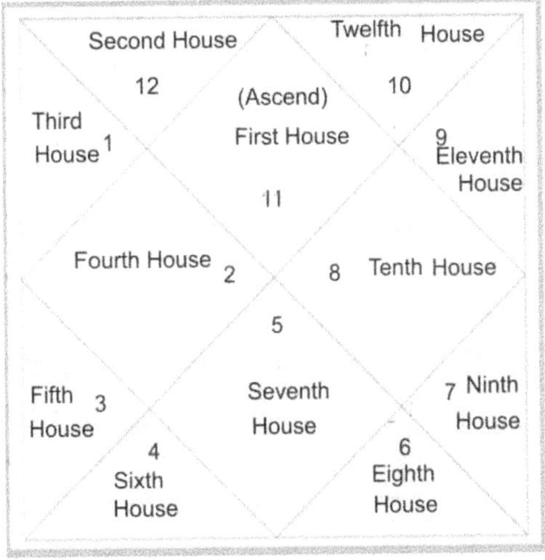

<u>**Zodiac Groups Sequences and their numbers in a Horoscope**</u>

Zodiac Group	Their No's
Aries	1
Taurus	2
Gemini	3
Cancer	4
Leo	5
Virgo	6
Libra	7
Scorpio	8
Sagittarius	9
Capricorns	10
Aquarius	11
Pisces	12

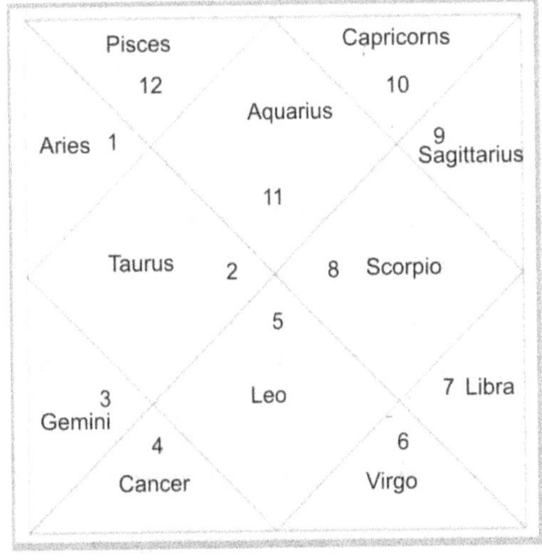

Pisces
12
Capricorns
10
Aquarius
Aries 1
9
Sagittarius
11
Taurus 2
8 Scorpio
5
3
Gemini
Leo
7 Libra
4
Cancer
6
Virgo

<u>**Planets and their sights on various houses**</u>

<u>**Planets**</u>	<u>**Full Sights**</u>
Sun	Seventh
Moon	Seventh
Venus	Seventh
Mercury	Seventh
Jupiter	Fifth, Seventh & Ninth
Saturn	Third, Seventh & Tenth
Marsh	Fourth, Seventh & Eight
Rahu	Fifth, Seventh & Ninth
Ketu	Fifth, Seventh & Ninth

Suppose the planet "Sun" be in zodiac group "Gemini" (Chart-2), then as per the Chart-1, it will be in "fifth' house. Now including the Fifth house, the seventh house from the fifth house is the "Eleventh house (zodiac group-Sagittarius") .Suppose in Eleventh house(Sagittarius zodiac group),planet "Jupiter" be there, then "Full Seventh Sight" of "Sun" will be on the planet "Jupiter". It is to be noted here that "Full seventh Sight" of "Jupiter" will also on the planet "Sun".

If the planet "Moon" be in zodiac group "Leo" (Chart-2),then as per the Chart-1, It will be in "Seventh" house. Now including the seventh house, seventh house from the seventh house is the "First House(Zodiac group

14

"Aquarius"). Suppose the planet Saturn" be in the first house, then "Seventh full sight" of "Moon" will be on the planet "Saturn" .It is to be noted that full Seventh sight of "Saturn" will also be on the "Planet-Moon".

Likewise the full seventh sights of the planets-Mercury and Venus will be.

If the planet "Marsh" be positioned in zodiac group-"Virgo" (Chart-2),then as per the Chart-1, it will be in the Eight house. Now Marsh has Fourth, Seventh and Eighth full sights. The fourth house from "Virgo" zodiac group is "Sagittarius". If the planet " Venus" be in the Sagittarius zodiac group, then fourth full sight of Marsh will be on Venus .Now let us assume that the planet "Mercury" be in zodiac group "Pisces" (2nd House, as per Chart-1),then from zodiac group "Virgo", it is in seventh house from Virgo. So now full seventh sight of Marsh will be on "Mercury". As Marsh is also at the seventh house from "Mercury, so full seventh sight of Mercury will also be on Marsh. If the planet "Jupiter" be in zodiac group-"Aries", eighth house from Virgo zodiac group, then full eighth sight of Marsh will be on "Jupiter".

If the planet "Jupiter" be in "Sagittarius" zodiac group, then as per the Chart-1, it is in the eleventh house. Jupiter has fifth, Seventh and ninth full sights. If Planet Moon be in "Aries" zodiac group, then full fifth sight of Jupiter will be on Moon. If the planet Venus be in zodiac group-"Gemini", then from Sagittarius zodiac group, it is in the seventh house, and so seventh full sight of Jupiter will be on Venus. As the planet Jupiter is at seventh house from the Gemini zodiac group, so full seventh sight of Venus will also be on the planet Jupiter. If the planet "Mercury" be in "Leo" zodiac group, then as per Chart-1, it is in the ninth house from the planet Jupiter and so full ninth sight of Jupiter will be on the planet Mercury.

Like wise are the full fifth, Seventh and Ninth sights of planets Rahu and Ketu.

If the planet "Saturn" be in zodiac group" Libra' , it is in the ninth house as per the Chart-1.Saturn has third, seventh and tenth full sights .If the planet "Moon" be in "Sagittarius' zodiac group, then it is in the third house from Libra and so third full sight of Saturn will be on "Moon". If the planet "Marsh" be in zodiac group-"Aries", then Marsh is at seventh house from Saturn and so full seventh sight of Saturn will be on Marsh. As Saturn is also at seventh house from Aries zodiac group, so full seventh sight of Marsh will be on Saturn. Now if the planet Venus be in the zodiac group "Cancer", then as per the Chart-1, it is in the tenth house from Libra zodiac group and so full tenth sight of Saturn will be on Venus.

Chapter 3

Date wise spreading analysis of Covid-19 Virus

On 15th Jan. 2020, Sun moved into Capricorns zodiac group .

Planetary   position on 15th jan. 2020 (As per Indian Astrology)----

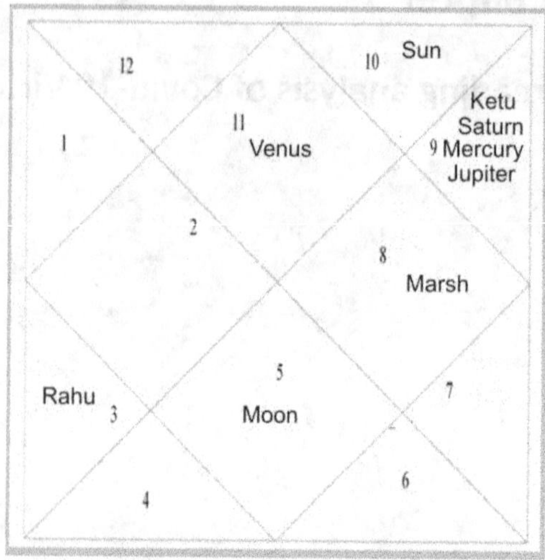

As the planets Jupiter and Mercury were still under the effects of Rahu, ketu, and Saturn and the ninth sight of Rahu and fourth sight of Marsh were on Venus, so Covid-19 infection was going on.

On 21st Jan. 2020, Mercury moved into Capricorns zodiac group

<u>**Planetary   position on 21st jan. 2020 (As per Indian Astrology)----**</u>

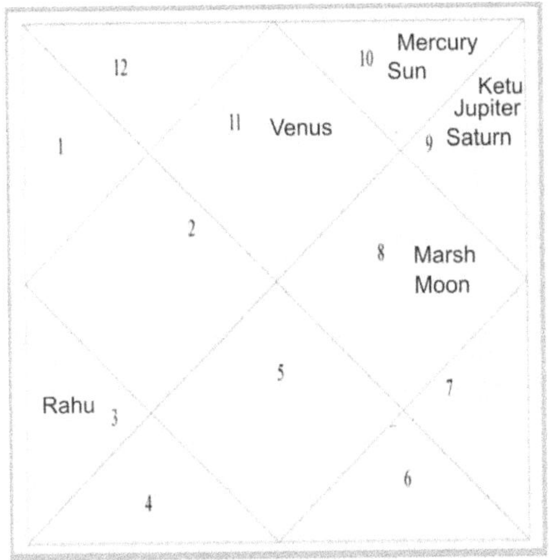

The planet Moon was under the effect of Marsh, Jupiter was under the effects of Saturn, Rahu and Ketu. Mercury was under the effect of Sun while ninth full sight of Rahu and fourth full sight of Marsh were on Venus. As all the four soft planets Moon, Jupiter, Mercury and Venus were under the effects of rough planets, so Covid-19 cases were increasing.

On 25th Jan. 2020, the planet Saturn entered into Capricorns zodiac group.

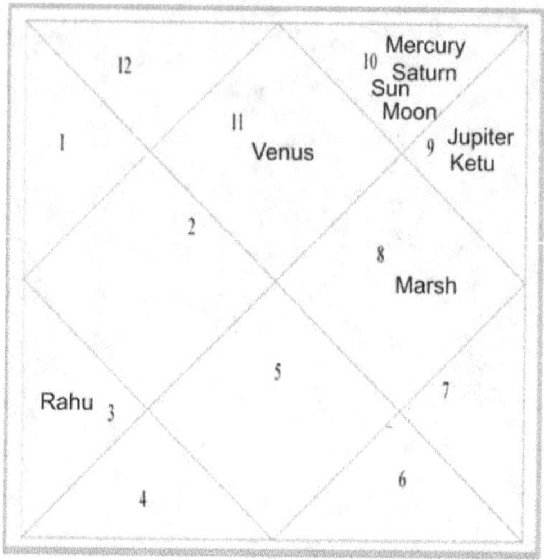

Now the planet Jupiter was under the effects of Rahu and Ketu, Mercury and Moon were under the effects of Sun and Saturn. Full fourth sights of Marsh and ninth sight of Rahu were on Venus. As all the four soft planets were under the effect of rough planets, So the Covid-19 cases were increasing.

On 31st Jan. 2020,Mercury moved into Aquarius zodiac group.

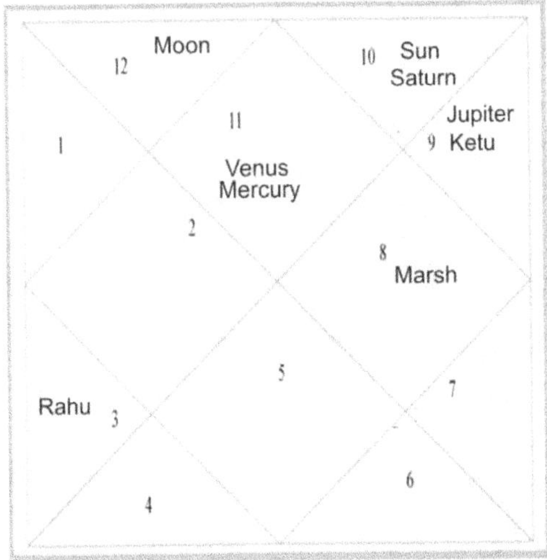

Now the planet Jupiter was under the effects of Rahu and Ketu .Fourth full sight of Marsh and ninth full sight of Rahu were on Venus and Mercury .Third sight of Saturn was an Moon. As still all the four soft planets were under the effects of rough planets So Covid-19 cases were go on increasing.

On 3ʳᵈ Feb. 2020, Venus entered into Pisces zodiac group.

<u>**Planetary   position on 3rd Feb. 2020 (As per Indian Astrology)----**</u>

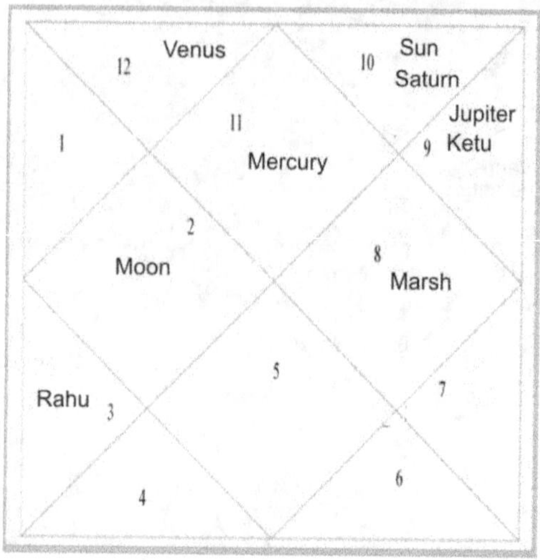

Now Jupiter was under the effects of Rahu and Ketu. Full fourth sight of Marsh and Ninth sight of Rahu were on Mercury. Third sight of Saturn was on Venus. Full seventh sight of Marsh was on Moon. As all the four soft planets were under the effects of rough planets So Covid-19 cases were increasing.

On 8th Feb. 2020, Marsh entered into Sagittarius zodiac group.

<u>**Planetary   position on 8th Feb. 2020 (As per Indian Astrology)----**</u>

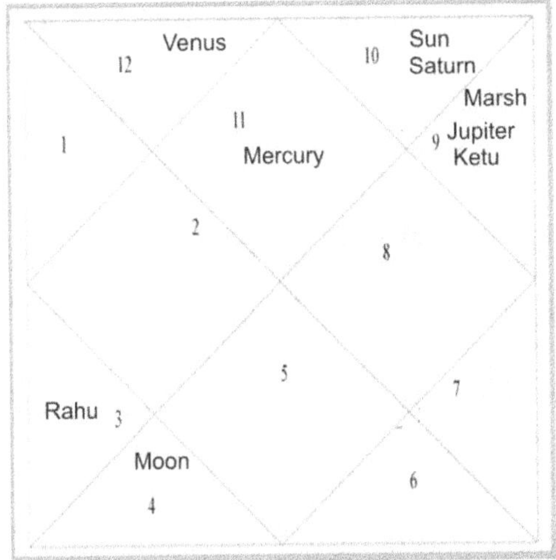

Now full seventh sight of Saturn and Sun were on Moon . Eighth full sight of Marsh was also on Moon.. Jupiter was under the effects of Rahu, ketu and Marsh. Full ninth sight of Rahu was on Mercury. Fourth sight of Marsh and third sight of Saturn were on Venus. As all the four soft planets were under the effects of rough planets So Covid-19 cases were go on increasing.

On 14th Feb. 2020, Sun moved into Aquarius.

<u>**Planetary   position on 14th Feb. 2020 (As per Indian Astrology)----**</u>

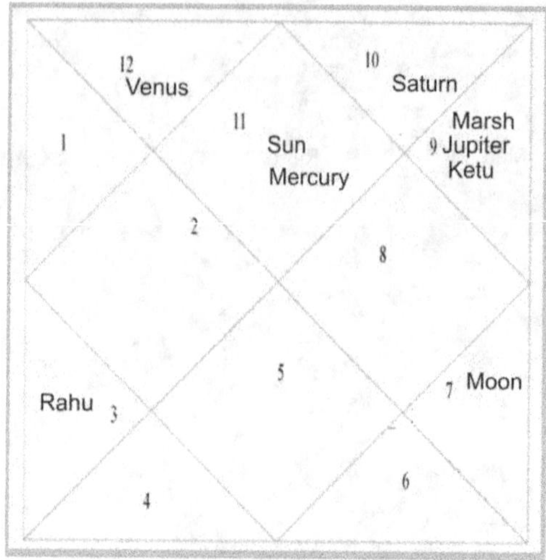

Now 10th full sight of Saturn and fifth full sight of Rahu were on Moon. Jupiter was under the effects of Rahu, ketu and Marsh. Mercury was under the effect of Sun. Ninth full sight of Rahu was also on Mercury. Fourth full sight of Marsh and third full sight of Saturn were on Venus. As all the four soft planets were under the effects of rough planets So Covid-19 cases were still go on increasing.

On 29th Feb. 2020, Venus entered into Aries zodiac group.

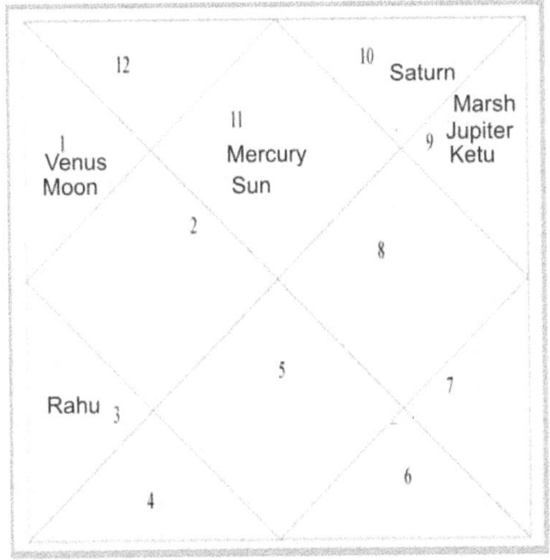

Now Jupiter was under the effects of Rahu, Ketu and Marsh.. Mercury was under the effect of Sun , The full ninth sight of Rahu was also on Mercury. The full fifth sight of Ketu was on Venus and Moon. As all the four soft planets were still under the effects of rough planets, so Covid-19 cases were increasing.

On 15th March 2020, Sun entered into Pisces zodiac group

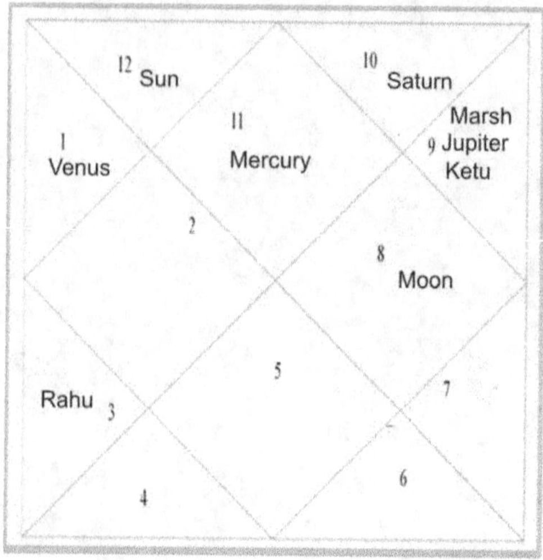

Now Jupiter was under the effects of Rahu, ketu and Marsh. The full ninth sight of Rahu was on Mercury. The full fifth sight of Ketu was on Venus. As except Moon, other three soft planets were under the effects of rough planets, so, Covid-19 cases were increasing.

On 23rd march 2020, Marsh entered into Capricorns zodiac group.

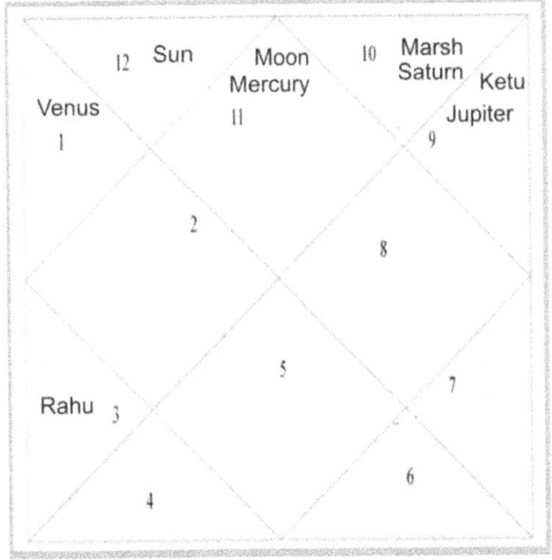

Now Jupiter was under the effects of Rahu and Ketu. Ninth sight of Rahu was on Mercury and Moon. Fifth sight of Ketu was on Venus. As all the four soft planets were under the effects of rough planets, so Covid-19 cases were go on increasing.

On 30th March 2020, Jupiter moved into Capricorns and Venus into Taurus zodiac group.

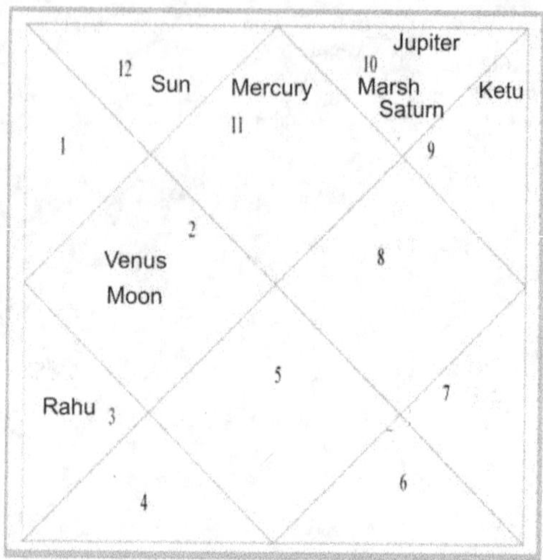

Now Jupiter was under the effects of Saturn and Marsh and full ninth sight of Rahu was on Mercury, But Venus and Moon were not under the effect of any rough planets. This combination of planets led the Covid-19 cases increasing.

On 7th April 2020, Mercury entered into Pisces zodiac group.

<u>**Planetary position on 7th April 2020 (As per Indian Astrology)----**</u>

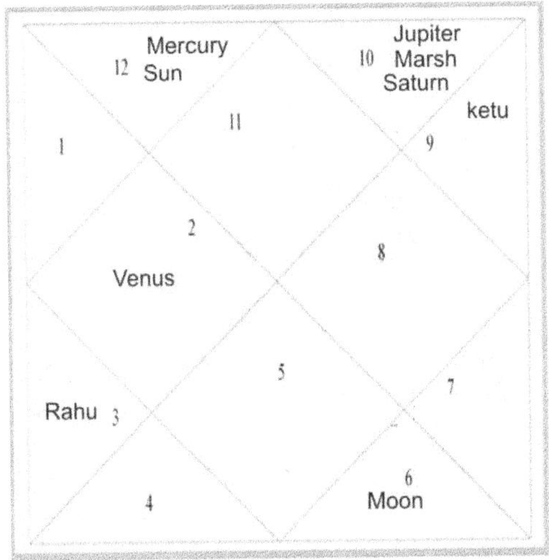

Now Venus was not under the effects of any rough planets, seventh full sight of Sun was on Moon. Jupiter was under the effects of Saturn and Marsh. Mercury was under the effect of Sun, full third sight of Saturn was on Mercury also. This combination of planets led the Covid-19 cases increasing.

On 13th April 2020, Sun moved into Aries zodiac group.

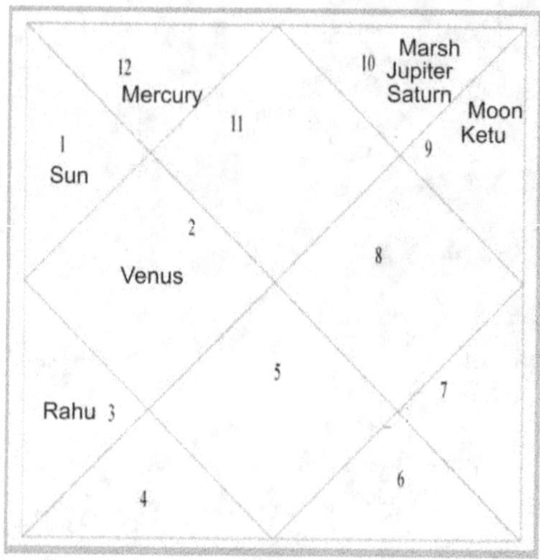

Now Moon was under the effects of Rahu and Ketu. Jupiter was under the effects of Saturn and Marsh. Third sight of Saturn was on Mercury. But as Venus was not under the effects of any rough planet so Covid-19 cases were decreasing.

On 25th April 2020, Mercury moved into Aries zodiac group.

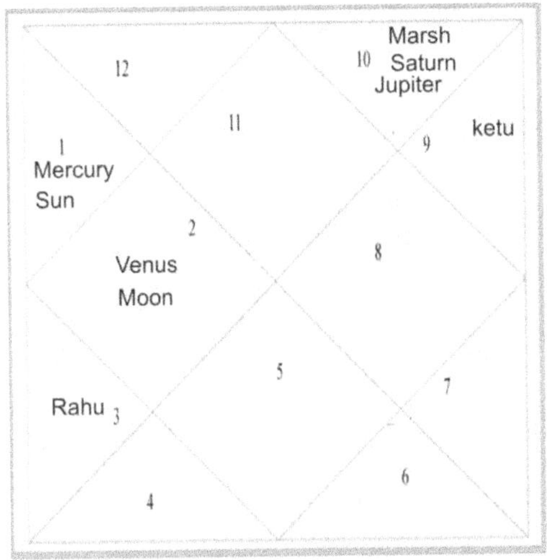

Now Venus and Moon were not under the effects of any rough planets, but Jupiter was under the effects of Saturn and Marsh. Mercury was under the effect of Sun. Full fifth sight of Ketu was on Jupiter. This combination of planets led to increase of Covid-19 cases.

On 4th May 2020, Marsh entered into Aquarius zodiac group.

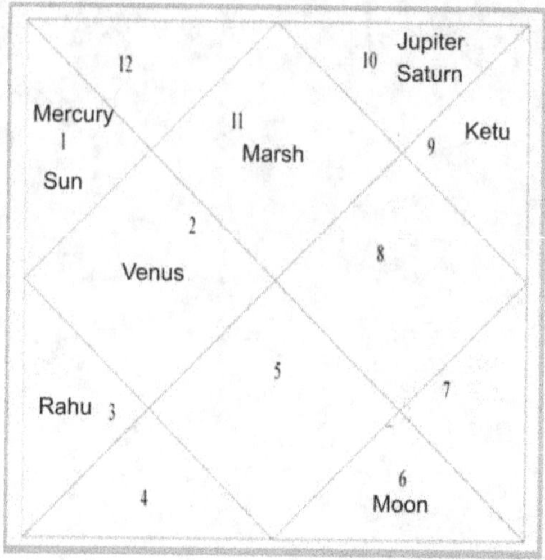

Now Jupiter was under the effect of Saturn. Mercury was under the effect of Sun ,full fifth sight of Ketu was also on Mercury and fourth full sight of Marsh was on Venus. As except Moon, other three soft planets were under the effects of rough planets, so Covid-19 cases were go on increasing.

On ninth May 1020, Mercury entered into Taurus zodiac group.

<u>**Planetary position on 9th May 2020 (As per Indian Astrology)----**</u>

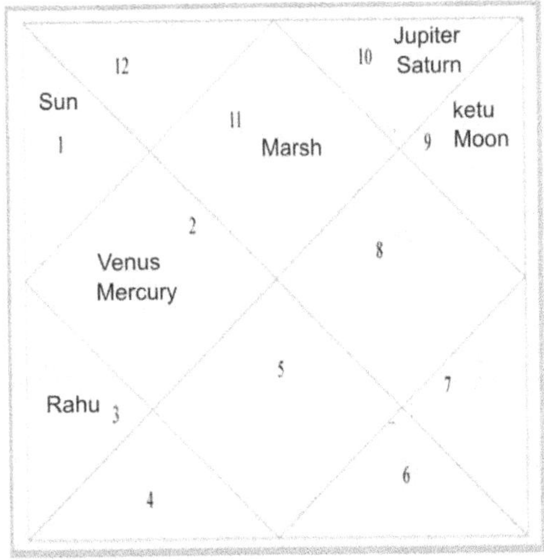

Now Moon was under the effects of Rahu and Ketu. Jupiter was under the effect of Saturn. Full fourth sight of Marsh was on Venus and Mercury. As all the four soft planets were under the effects of rough planets, so Covid-19 cases were increasing.

On 16th May 2020, Sun entered into Taurus zodiac group.

<u>**Planetary   position on 16th May 2020 (As per Indian Astrology)----**</u>

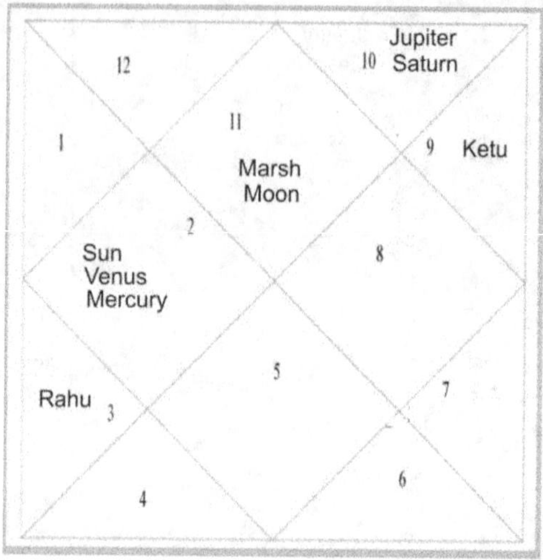

Now Jupiter was under the effect of Saturn. Moon was under the effect of Marsh. Full ninth sight of Rahu was on Moon. Venus and Mercury were under the effect of Sun. As all the four soft planets were under the effects of rough planets, so Covid-19 cases were increasing.

On 25th May 2020, Mercury moved into Gemini zodiac group.

34

<u>**Planetary   position on 25th May 2020 (As per Indian Astrology)----**</u>

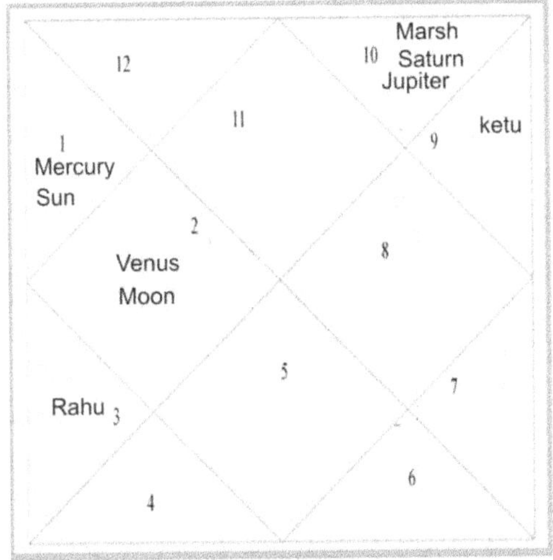

Now Mercury and Moon were under the effects of Rahu and Ketu. Jupiter was under the effect of Saturn. Venus was under the effect of Sun ,also fourth full sight of Marsh was on Venus. As all the four soft planets were under the effects of rough planets, so Covid-19 cases were increasing.

On 15th June 2020, Sun moved into Gemini zodiac group.

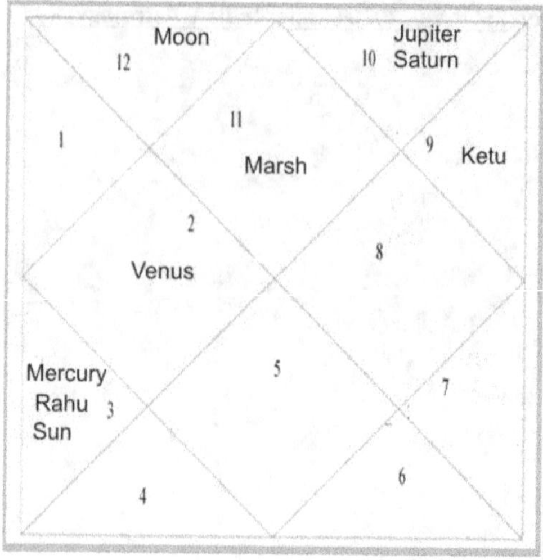

Now Mercury was under the effects of Rahu, Ketu and Sun. Jupiter was under the effect of Saturn. Third full sight of Saturn was on Moon and fourth full sight of Marsh was on Venus.

Once again, all the four soft planets were under the effects of rough planets, so the Covid-19 cases were increasing.

On 19th June 2020, Marsh moved into Pisces zodiac group.

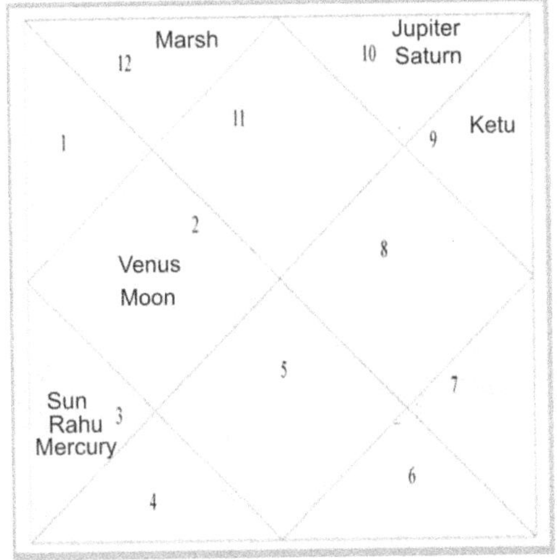

Now   Mercury was under the effects of Rahu, Ketu and Sun, further fourth full sight of Marsh was also on Mercury. Jupiter was under the effect of Saturn. But Venus and moon were not under the effect of any rough planets, So Covid-19 cases were decreasing.

On 30th June 2020, Jupiter entered into Sagittarius zodiac group with retarding motion.

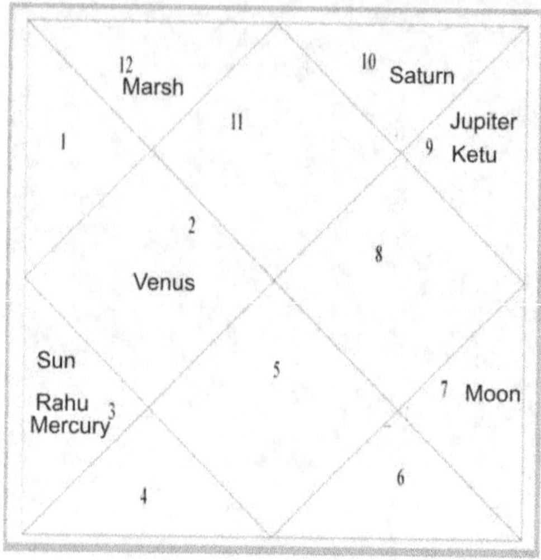

Now Mercury was under the effects of Rahu, ketu and Sun. Full fourth sight of Marsh was also on Mercury. Jupiter was under the effect of Rahu and ketu, full seventh sight of Sun was also on Jupiter. Full tenth sight of Saturn and eighth sight of Marsh were on Moon. But as Now Venus was not under the effects of any of the rough planets, So the Covid-19 cases were decreasing.

On 17th July 2020, Sun moved into Cancer zodiac group.

<u>**Planetary   position on 17th July 2020 (As per Indian Astrology)----**</u>

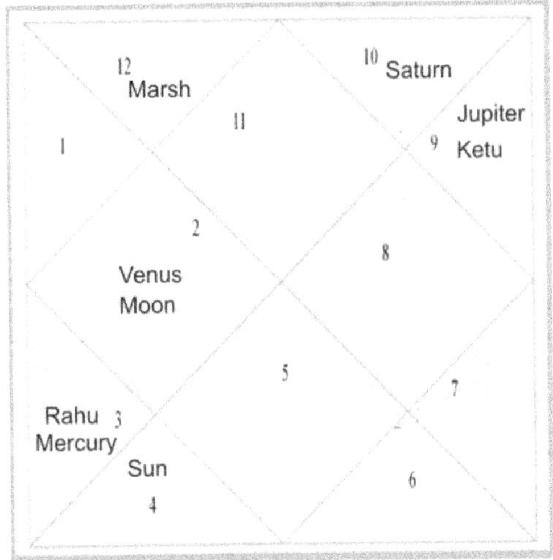

Now now Mercury was under the effects of Rahu and ketu, full fourth sight of Marsh was on Mercury. Jupiter was under the effects of Rahu and ketu. But as Venus and Moon were not under the effect of any of the rough planets, So the cases of Covid-19 were decreasing.

On 1st August 2020, Venus moved into Gemini zodiac group.

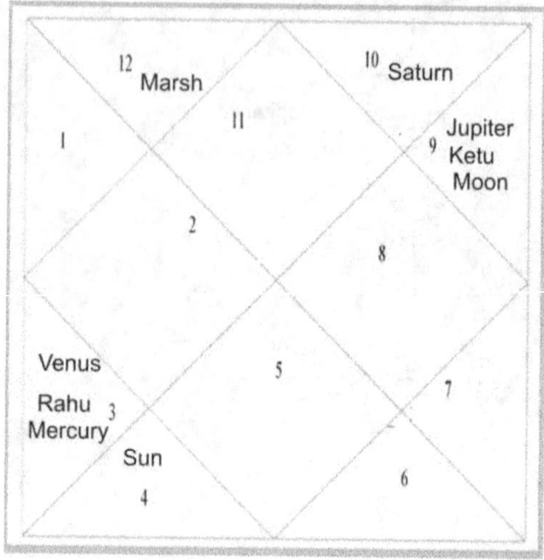

Now Venus and Mercury were under the effects of Rahu and Ketu. Full fourth sight of Marsh was also on Venus and Mercury. Jupiter and Moon were under the effects of Rahu and Ketu. As all the four soft planets were under the effects of rough planets, so the cases of Covid-19 started increasing.

On 2nd August 2020, Mercury moved into Cancer zodiac group.

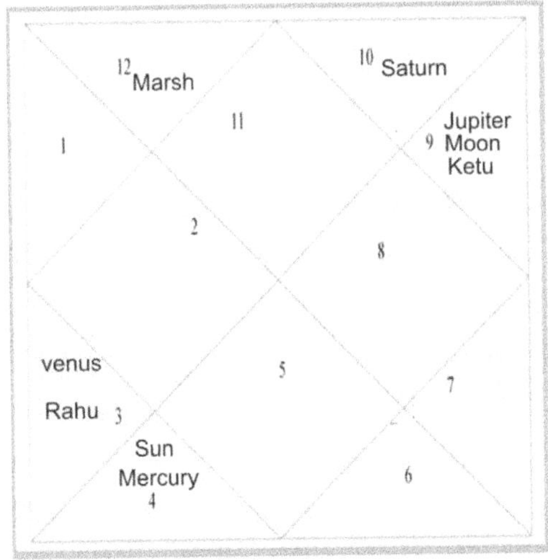

Now Venus was under the effects of Rahu and Ketu, Fourth full sight of Marsh was also on Venus. Mercury was under the effect of Sun. Seventh full sight of Saturn was also on Mercury. Jupiter and Moon were under the effects of Rahu and Ketu. As all the four soft planets were under the effects of rough planets so the cases of Covid-19 were increasing on.

On 17th August, Sun moved into Leo zodiac group and Marsh into Aries

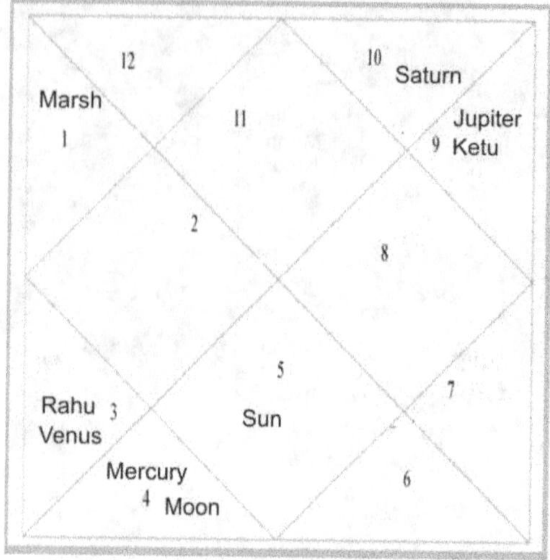

Now Venus was under the effect of Rahu and Ketu. Full seventh sight of Saturn and fourth sight of Marsh were on Mercury and Moon .Jupiter was under the effects of Rahu and Ketu. As all the four soft planets were under the effects of rough planets So Covid-19 cases were increasing on.

On 18th August 2020, Mercury moved into Leo zodiac group.

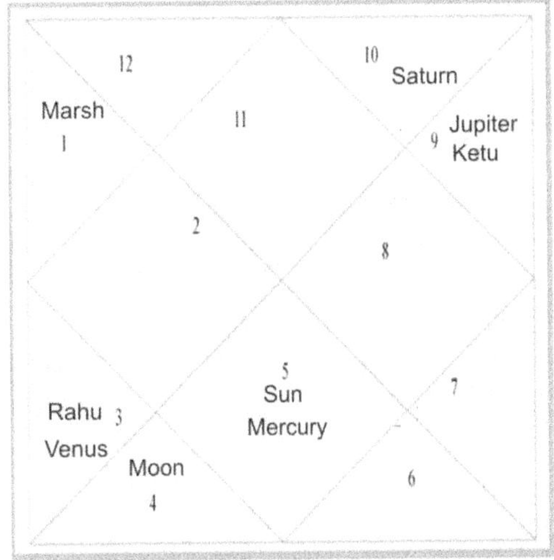

Now Venus was under the effects of Rahu and Ketu, Seventh sight of Saturn and fourth sight of Marsh were on Moon. Mercury was under the effect of Sun. Ninth full sight of Ketu was on Mercury. Jupiter was under the effects of Rahu and Ketu. As all the four soft planets were under the effects of rough planets, so Covid-19 effects were increasing on.

On 1st Sept. 2020, Venus moved into Cancer zodiac group.

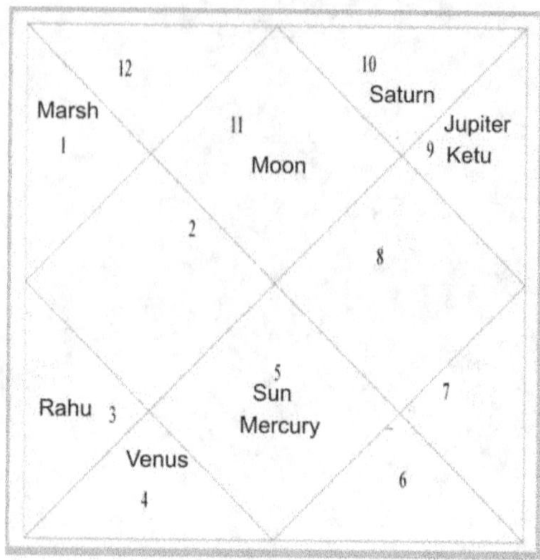

Now Full fourth sight of Marsh was on Venus. Mercury was under the effect of Sun .Full ninth sight of Ketu was also on Mercury. Full ninth sight of Rahu and full seventh of Sun were on Moon. Jupiter was under the effects of Rahu and Ketu. As all the four soft planets were under the effects of rough planets, so Covid-19 cases were increasing on.

On 3rd Sept. 2020, Mercury moved into Virgo zodiac group.

<u>**Planetary   position on 3rd September 2020 (As per Indian Astrology)—**</u>

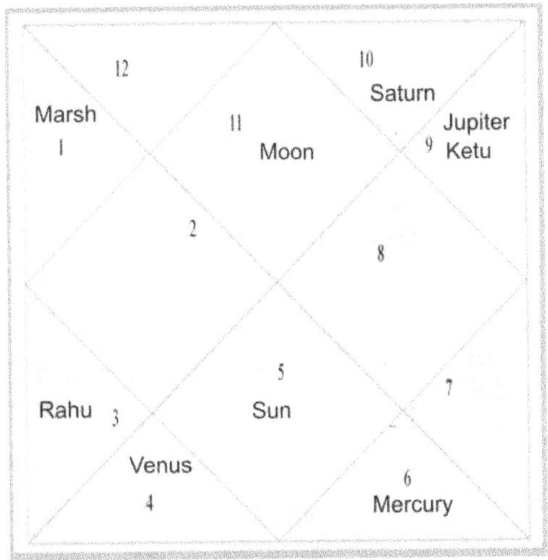

The full fourth sight of Marsh and seventh sight of Saturn were on Venus. Jupiter was under the effects of Rahu and Ketu. As Mercury was not under the effects of any rough planets, so Covid-19 cases started decreasing.

On 17th Sept. 2020, Sun moved into Virgo zodiac group.

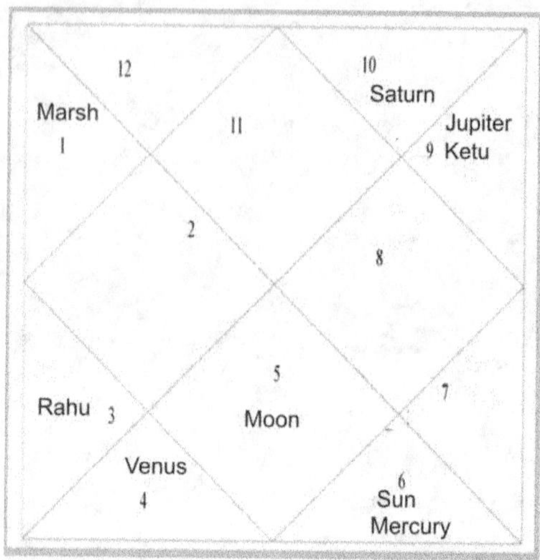

Now full seventh sight of Saturn and full fourth sight of Marsh were on Venus. Ninth sight of Ketu was on Moon, Mercury was under the effect of Sun and Jupiter was under the effect of Rahu and Ketu. As all the four soft planets were under the effects of rough planets, so Covid-19 cases were increasing.

On 22nd Sept. 2020, Mercury moved into Libra zodiac group

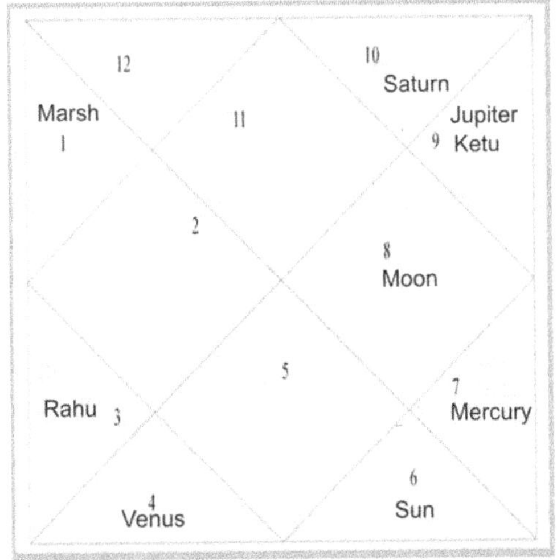

Now Full seventh sight of Saturn and full fourth sight of Marsh were on Venus. Full tenth sight of Saturn, Full seventh sight of Marsh and fifth sight of Rahu were on Mercury. Full eighth sight of Marsh was on Moon..Jupiter was under the effects of Rahu and Ketu. As all the four soft planets were under the effects of rough planets, so Covid-19 cases were go on increasing.

On 24th Sept. 2020, Rahu moved into Taurus and Ketu into Scorpio zodiac groups.

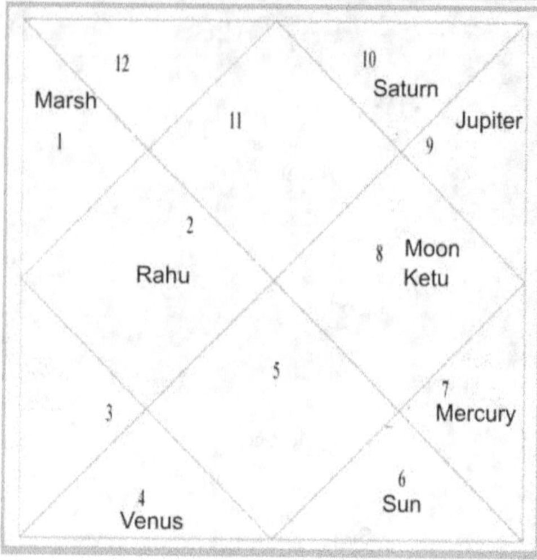

Now Full seventh sight of Saturn , fourth sight of Marsh and ninth sight of ketu were on Venus. Full tenth sight of Saturn and seventh sight of Marsh were on Mercury. Moon was under the effects of Rahu and Ketu. But as Jupiter was not under the effects of any of the rough planets, so Covid-19 cases started decreasing.

On 28th Sept. 2020, Venus entered into Leo zodiac group.

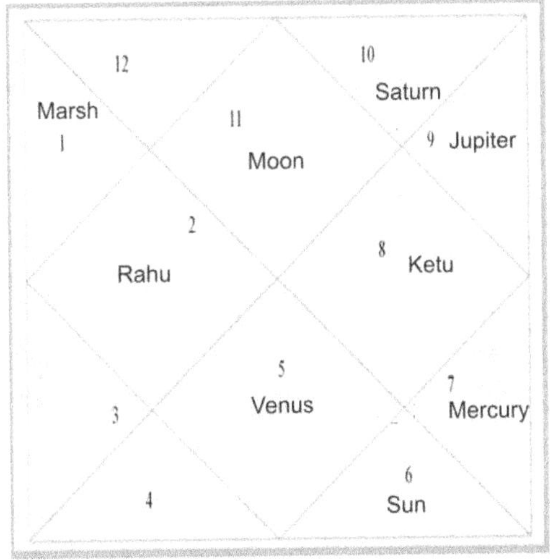

Now full tenth sight of Saturn and seventh sight of Marsh were on Mercury. But as Jupiter, moon and Venus were not under the effects of any of the rough planets, so Covid-19 cases started decreasing drastically.

On 5th October 2020, Marsh moved into Pisces zodiac group with retarding motion.

<u>**Planetary   position on 5th October 2020 (As per Indian Astrology)-**</u>

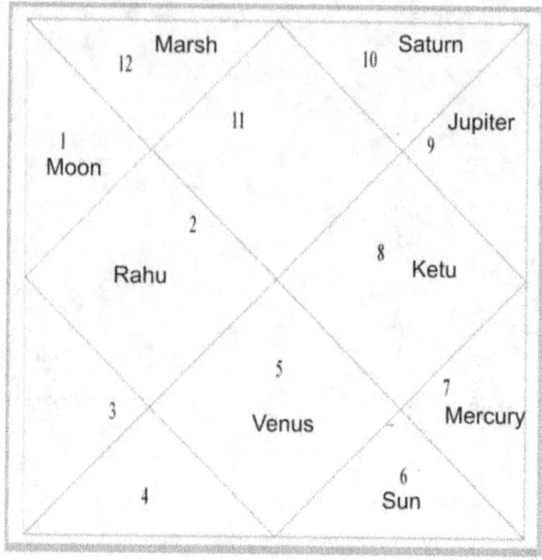

Now full tenth sight of Saturn and eighth sight of Marsh were on Mercury. As soft planets Moon, Venus and Jupiter were not under the effects of any of the rough planets, so decrease in Covid-19 cases were going on.

On 18th October 2020, Sun moved into Libra zodiac group.

<u>**Planetary   position on 18th October 2020 (As per Indian Astrology)----**</u>

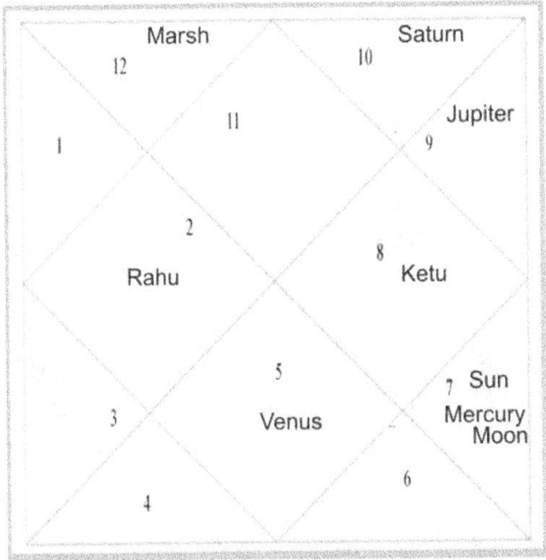

Now Mercury and Moon were under the effects of Sun, full tenth sight of Saturn and eighth sight of Marsh were on Mercury and Moon. But as Jupiter and Venus were not under the effects of any of the rough planets, so decrease in Covid-19 cases were going on.

On 24th October 2020, Venus entered into Virgo zodiac group.

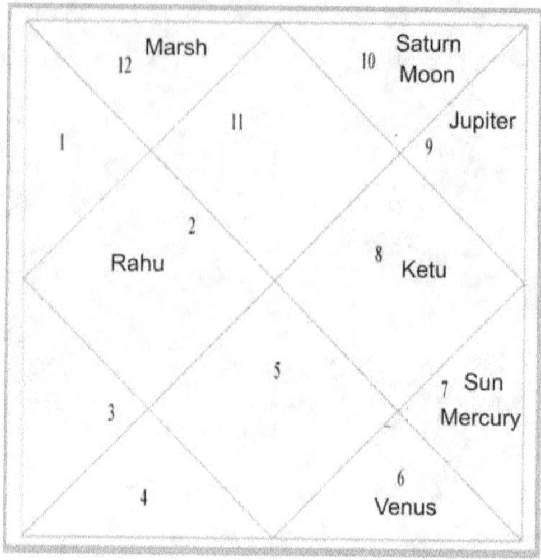

Now full seventh sight of Marsh was on Venus, fifth sight of Rahu was also on Venus. Mercury was under the effect of Sun. Full tenth sight of Saturn and eighth sight of Marsh were on Mercury. Moon was under the effect of Saturn. full ninth sight of Rahu was on Moon. But as Jupiter was not under the effect of any of the rough planets, so decrease in Covid-19 cases were going on.

On 17th Nov. 2020, Sun entered into Scorpio and Venus into Libra zodiac groups.

<u>**Planetary   position on 17th Nov.   2020 (As per Indian Astrology)----**</u>

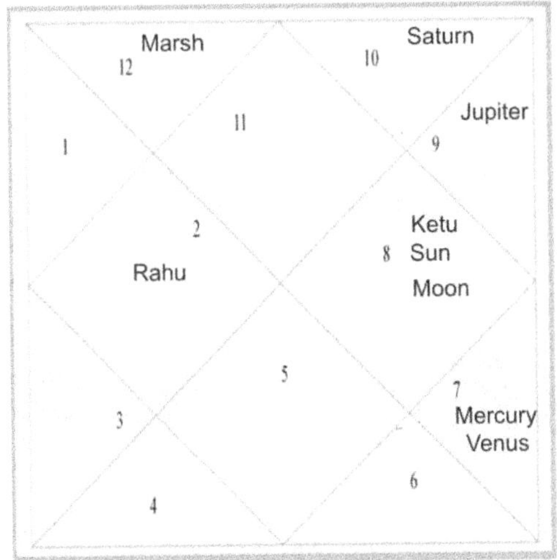

Now full tenth sight of Saturn and eighth sight of Marsh were on Venus and Mercury. Moon was under the effects of Rahu, Ketu and Sun. But as Jupiter was not under the effect of any of the rough planets, so Covid-19 cases were still decreasing.

On 21st Nov. 2020, Jupiter entered into Capricorns zodiac group.

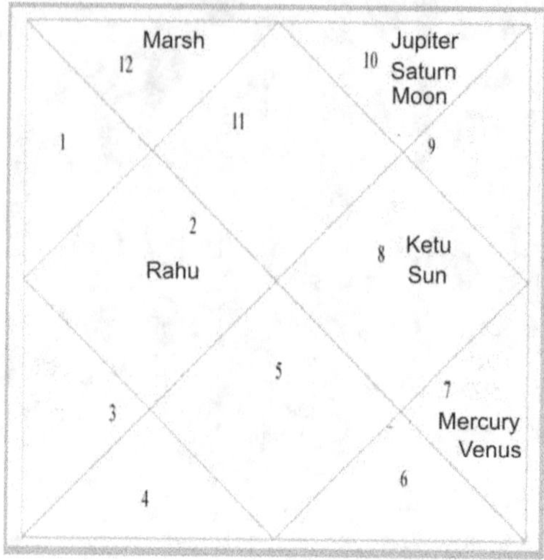

Now full tenth sight of Saturn was on Venus and Mercury, full eighth sight of Marsh was on Venus and Mercury. Jupiter was under the effect of Saturn. Further full ninth sight of Rahu was also on Jupiter and Moon. As all the four soft planets were under the effects of rough planets, so cases of Covid-19 cases had been increasing again.

On 29th Nov. 2020, Mercury moved into Scorpio zodiac group.

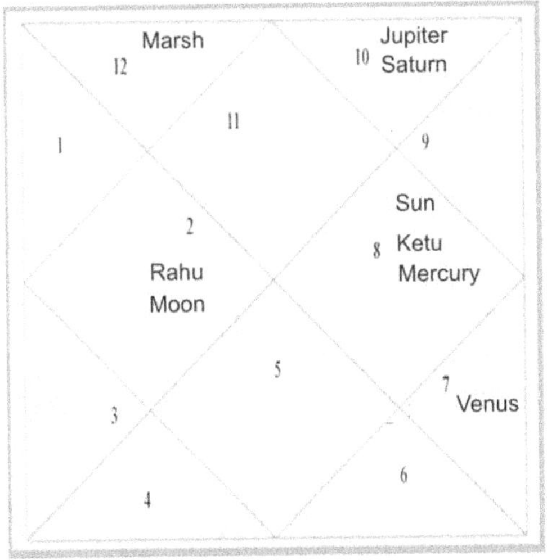

Now, Moon was under the effects of Rahu and Ketu, full seventh sight of Sun was also on Moon. Full tenth sight of Saturn and eighth sight of Marsh was on Venus. Mercury was under the effects of Rahu, Ketu and Sun. Jupiter was under the effect of Saturn. Full ninth sight of Rahu was also on Jupiter, as all the four soft planets were under the effects of rough planets, so Covid-19 cases were go on increasing.

On 11th Dec. 2020, Venus entered into Scorpio zodiac group.

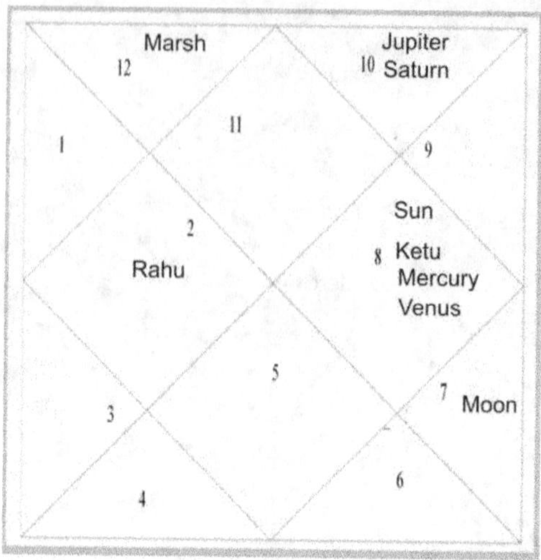

Now Venus and Mercury were under the effects of Rahu, Ketu and Sun, full tenth sight of Saturn and eighth sight of Marsh were on Moon. Jupiter was under the effect of Saturn, full ninth sight of Rahu was also on Jupiter. Once again all the four soft planets were under the effects of rough planets, so Covid-19 cases had been increasing on.

On 17th Dec. 2020, Sun moved into Sagittarius zodiac group.

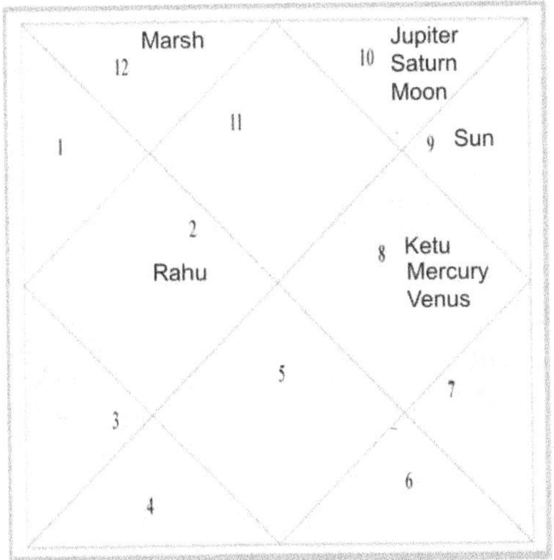

Now Venus and Mercury were under the effects of Rahu and Ketu. Jupiter and Moon were under the effect of Saturn. Full ninth sight of Rahu was on Jupiter and moon. As still all the four soft planets were under the effects of rough planets, so Covid-19 cases were go on increasing.

On 18th Dec. 2020, Mercury moved into Sagittarius zodiac group.

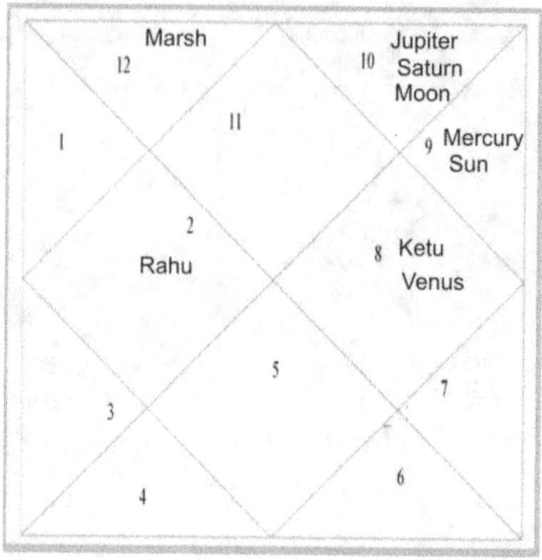

Now Venus was under the effect of Rahu and Ketu. Mercury was under the effect of Sun. Moon and Jupiter were under the effect of Saturn. Further full ninth sight of Rahu was on Jupiter and Moon. As still all the four soft planets were under the effects of rough planets, so Covid-19 cases were going increasing on.

On 25th Dec. 2020, Marsh moved into Aries zodiac group.

<u>**Planetary position on 25th December 2020 (As per Indian Astrology)-**</u>

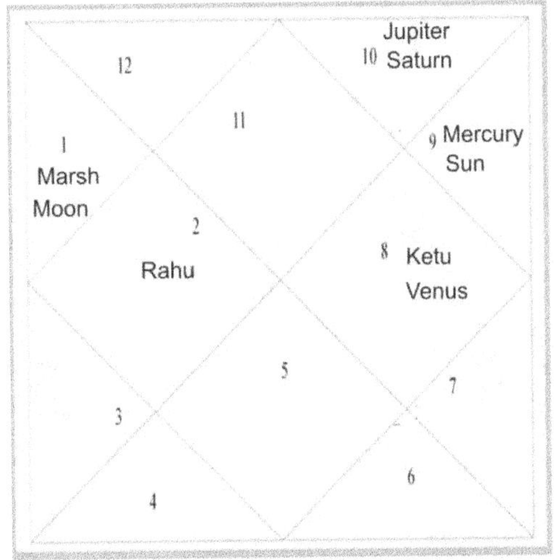

Now Moon was under the effect of Marsh. Venus was under the effects of Rahu and ketu. Full eighth sight of Marsh was on Venus. Mercury was under the effect of Sun. Jupiter was under the effect of Saturn. Also the full ninth sight of Rahu was on Jupiter. As still all the four soft planets were under the effects of rough planets, so Covid-19 cases were go on increasing.

On 4th Jan. 2020 Venus will move into Sagittarius and on 5th Jan. 2021 Mercury will move into Capricorns zodiac group.

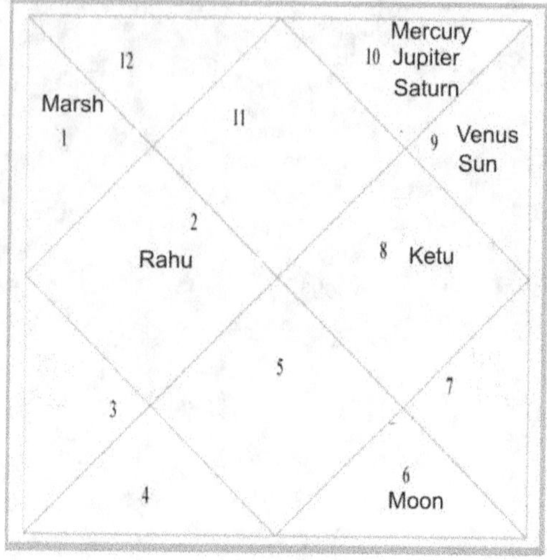

Now full fifth sight of Rahu will be on Moon. Venus will be under the effect of Sun. Jupiter and Mercury will be under the effect of Saturn. Full ninth sight of Rahu will also be on Jupiter and Mercury. As all the four soft planets will be under the effects of rough planets, so Covid-19 infections will go on increasing.

On 15th Jan. 2021 Sun will move into Capricorns zodiac group.

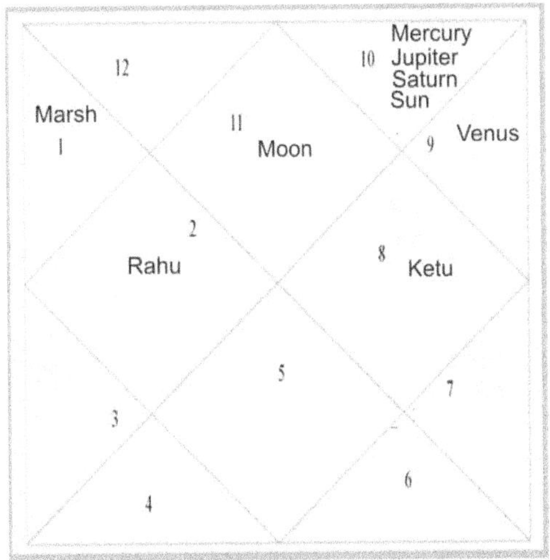

Now Jupiter and Mercury will be under the effects of Saturn and Sun. Full ninth sight of Rahu will also on Jupiter and Mercury. But as Venus and Moon will not be under the effects of any rough planets, so Covid-19 cases will start decreasing.

On 26th Jan. 2021, Mercury will move   into Aquarius and on 28th jan. 2021 Venus will move into Capricorns zodiac group.

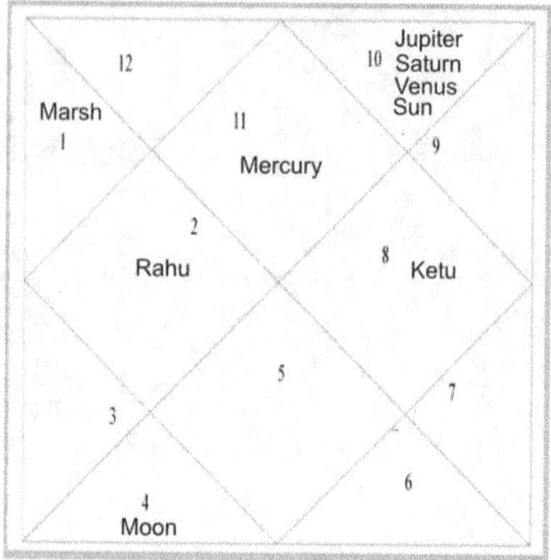

Now full fourth sight of Marsh , Full seventh sights of Sun and Saturn will be on Moon. Venus and Jupiter will be under the effects of Sun and Saturn. Full ninth sight of Rahu will be on Jupiter and Venus. But as Mercury will not be under the effect of any rough planets, so Covid-19 cases will go on decreasing.

On 6th Feb. 2021, Mercury will move into Capricorns zodiac group with retarding motion.

<u>**Planetary   position on 6th Feb. 2021 (As per Indian Astrology)----**</u>

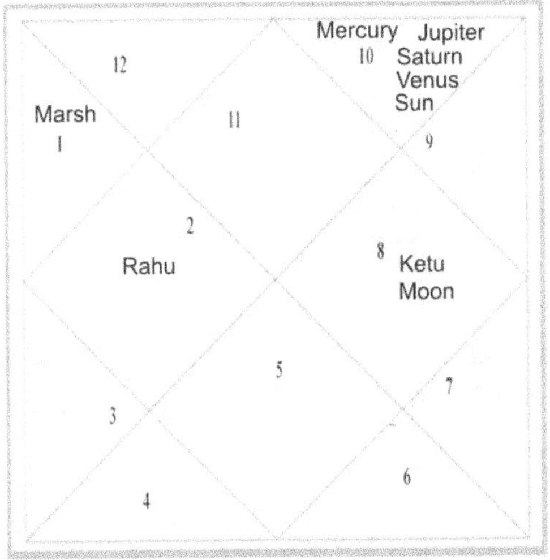

Now moon will be under the effects of Rahu and Ketu, full eighth sight of Marsh will be on Moon. Jupiter, Venus and Mercury will be under the effects of Saturn and Sun. Full ninth sight of Rahu will also be on Jupiter, Mercury and Venus. As all the four soft planets will be under the effects of rough planets, so Covid-19 cases will go on increasing.

On 13th Feb. 2021, Sun will move into Aquarius zodiac group.

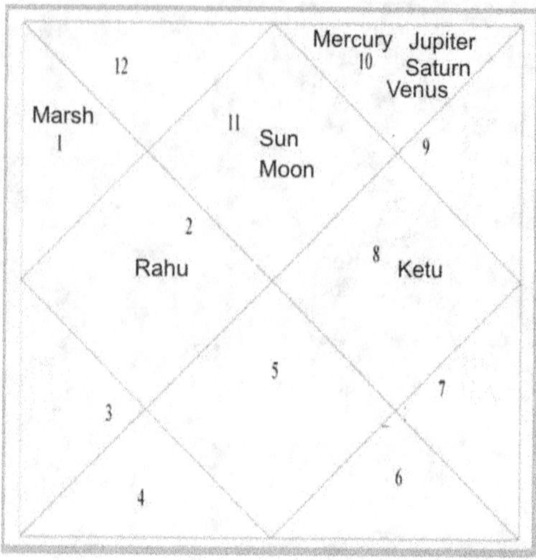

Now Moon will be under the effect of Sun. Jupiter, Mercury and Venus will be under the effects of Saturn. Full ninth sight of Rahu will also be on Jupiter, Mercury and Venus. As all the four soft planets will be under the effects of rough planets, so Covid-19 cases will go on increasing.

On 21st Feb. 2021, Venus will move into Aquarius zodiac group.

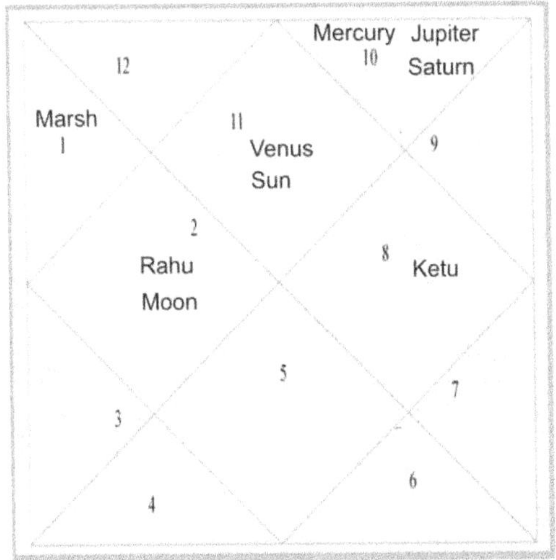

Now Moon will be under the effect of Rahu and Ketu, Jupiter and Mercury will be under the effect of Saturn. Full ninth sight of Rahu will be on Jupiter and Mercury. Venus will be under the effect of Sun. As all the four soft planets are under the effects of rough planets, so Covid-19 cases will go on increasing.

On 22nd Feb. 2021, Marsh will enter into Taurus zodiac group.

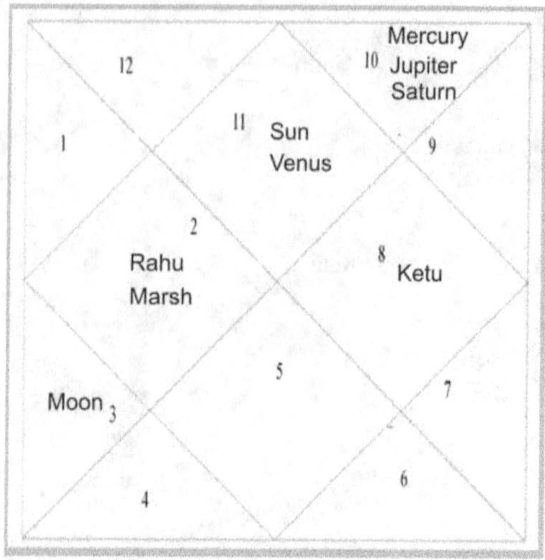

Now Jupiter and Mercury will be under the effect of Saturn. Full ninth sight of Rahu will be on Jupiter and Mercury. Venus will be under the effect of Sun. As except Moon, all other three soft planets will be under the effects of rough planets, so Covid-19 case will be moving as such.

On 12th March 2021, Mercury will move into Aquarius zodiac group.

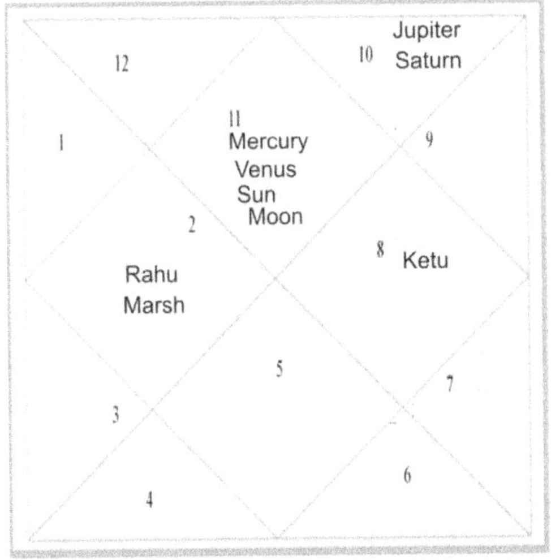

Now Jupiter will be under the effect of Saturn. Full ninth sight of Rahu will also be on Jupiter. Mercury, Venus and Moon will be under the effect of Sun. As all the four soft planets will be under the effects of rough planets, so Covid-19 cases will go on increasing.

On 15th March 2021, Sun will move into Pisces zodiac group.

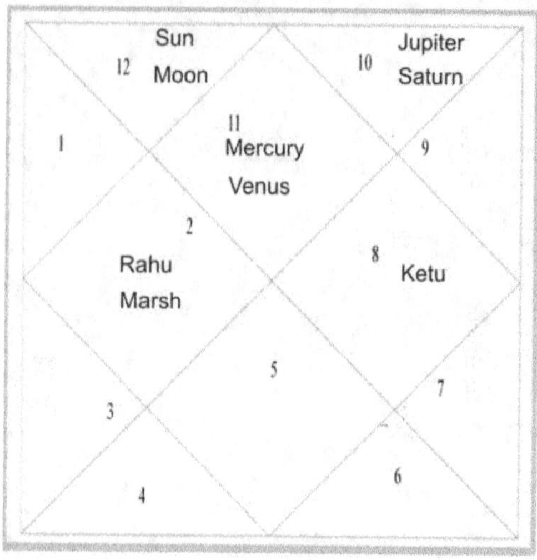

Now Jupiter will be under the effect of Saturn. Full ninth sight of Rahu will also be on Jupiter. Moon will be under the effect of Sun. Full fifth sight of Ketu will also be on Moon. But as soft planets Venus and Mercury will not be under the effects of any of the rough planets, so Covid-19 cases will start decreasing.

On 17th March 2021 , Venus will enter into Pisces zodiac group.

<u>**Planetary position on 17th March 2021 (As per Indian Astrology)—**</u>

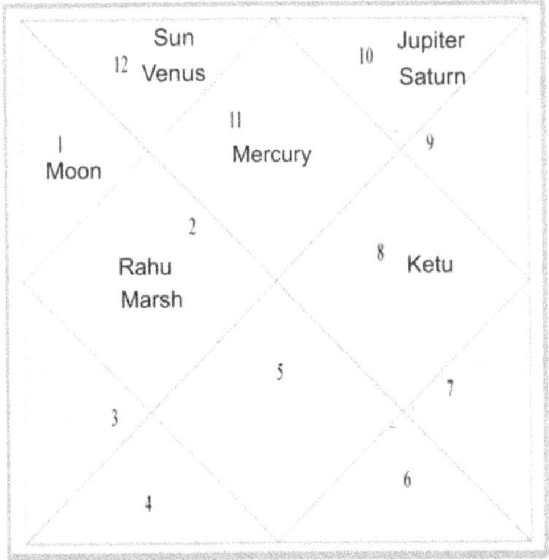

Now Jupiter will be under the effect of Saturn, full ninth sight of Rahu will also be on Jupiter. Venus will be under the effect of Sun, full fifth sight of Ketu and third sight of Saturn will also be on Venus. But as soft planets Mercury and Moon are not under the effects of any of the rough planets, so Covid-19 cases will still go on decreasing.

On 2nd April 2021, Mercury will move into Pisces zodiac group.

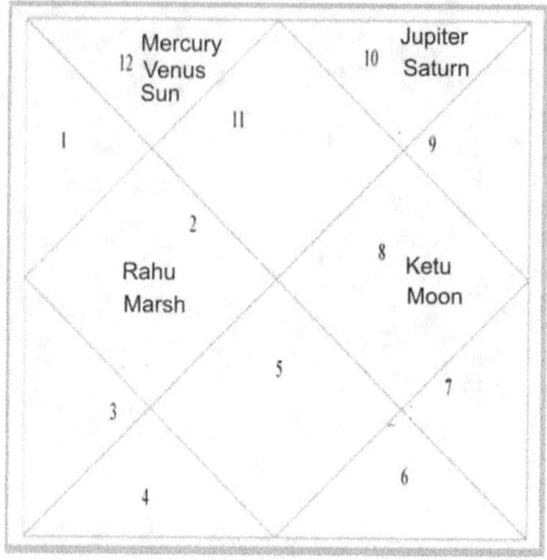

Now Jupiter will be under the effect of Saturn, full ninth sight of Rahu will also be on Jupiter. Moon will be under the effects of Rahu and Ketu, full seventh sight of Marsh will also be on Moon. Venus and Mercury will be under the effect of Sun .Fifth full sight of Ketu and third sight of Saturn will also be on Venus and Mercury. As all the four soft planets will be under the effects of rough planets, so Covid-19 cases will go on increasing.

On 6th April 2021, Jupiter will move into Aquarius zodiac group.

<u>**Planetary position on 6th April 2021 (As per Indian Astrology)----**</u>

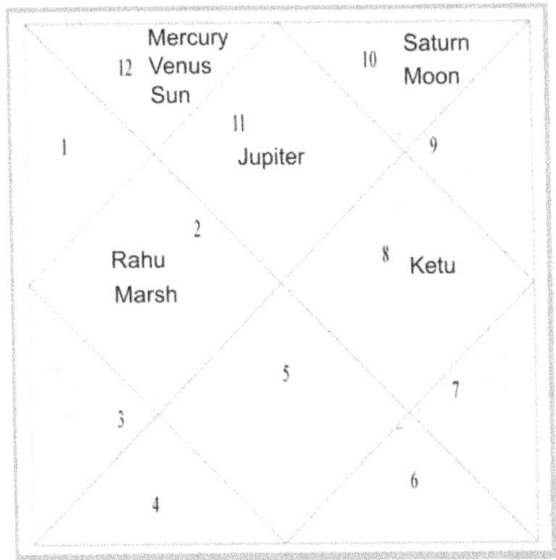

Now Moon will be under the effect of Saturn, full ninth sight of Rahu will also be on Moon. Venus and Mercury will be under the effect of Sun. Full third sight of Saturn will also be on Venus and Mercury. But as Jupiter will not be under the effect of any of the rough planets, so Covid-19 cases will go on decreasing.

On 10th April 2021, Venus will move into Pisces zodiac group.

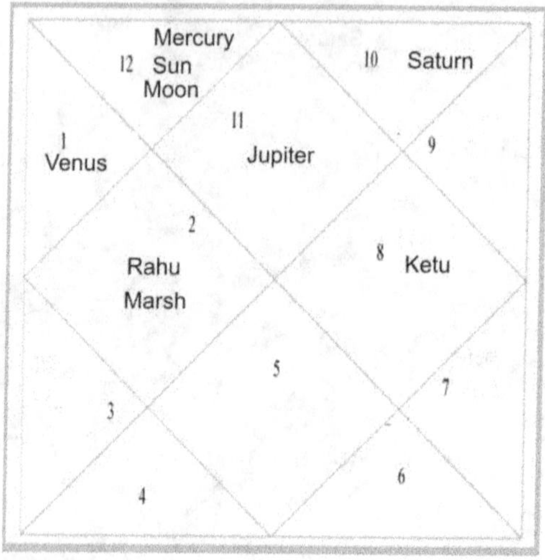

Now Mercury and Moon will be under the effect of Sun. Full third sight of Saturn will also be on Mercury and Moon. But as Venus and Jupiter will not be under the effects of any of the rough planets, so Covid-19 cases will further go on decreasing.

On 14th April 2021, Sun will move into Aries and Marsh into Gemini zodiac group.

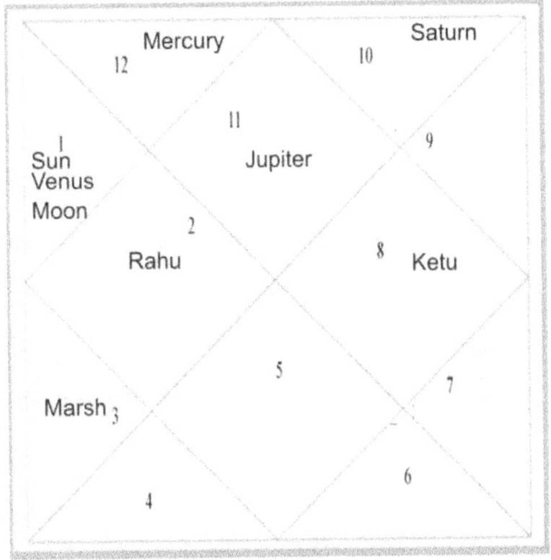

Now full third sight of Saturn will be on Mercury, full fifth sight of Ketu
will also be on Mercury. Venus and Moon will be under the effect of Sun.
However as Jupiter will not be under the effect of any rough planet, so
Covid-19 cases will go on decreasing.

On 17th April 2021, Mercury will move into Aries zodiac group.

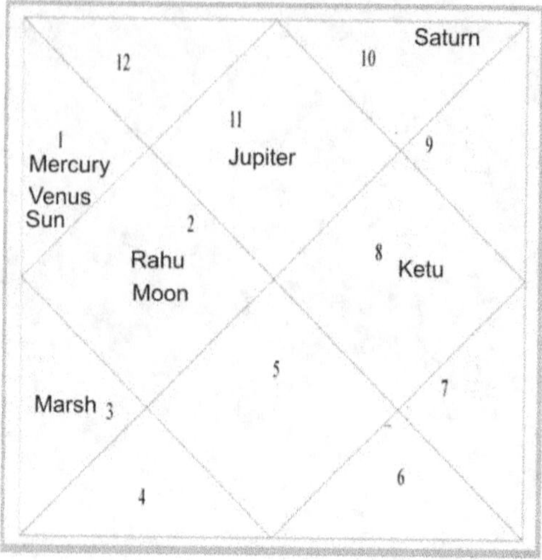

Now Venus and Mercury will be under the effect of Sun. Moon will be under the effect of Rahu and Ketu. But as Jupiter will not be under the effect of any of the rough planet, so Covid-19 cases will go on decreasing.

On 1st May 2021, Mercury will move into Taurus zodiac group.

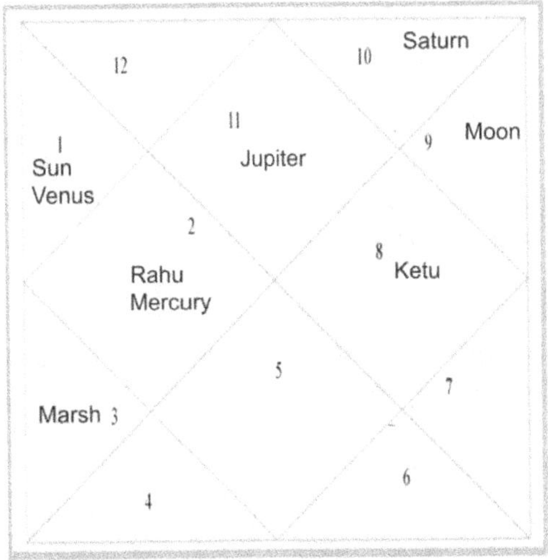

Now full seventh sight of Marsh will be on Moon. Venus will be under the effect of Sun. Mercury will be under the effect of Rahu and Ketu. However as Jupiter will not be under the effect of any rough planet, so Covid-19 cases will go on decreasing.

On 5th May 2021, Venus will move into Taurus zodiac group.

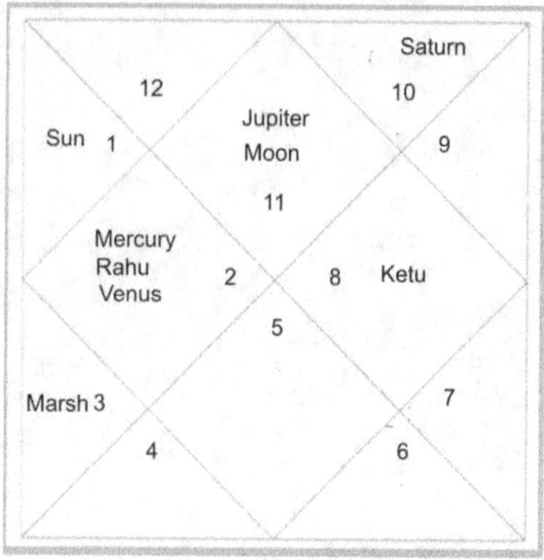

Now Mercury and Venus will be under the effects of Rahu and Ketu. But as Jupiter and Moon will not be under the effect of any rough planet, so Covid-19 cases will go on decreasing.

On 15th May 2021, Sun will move into Taurus zodiac group.

<u>**Planetary position on 15th May 2021 (As per Indian Astrology)----**</u>

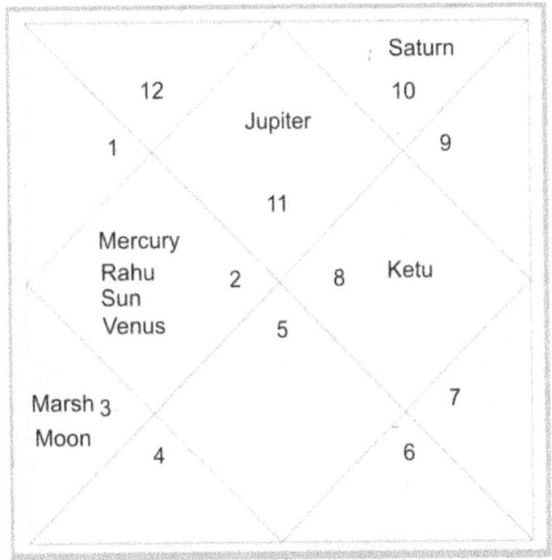

Now Moon will be under the effect of Marsh. Mercury and Venus will be under the effects of Rahu, Ketu and Sun. But as Jupiter will not be under the effect of any rough planet, so Covid-19 cases will go on decreasing.

On 27th May 2021, Mercury will move into Gemini zodiac group

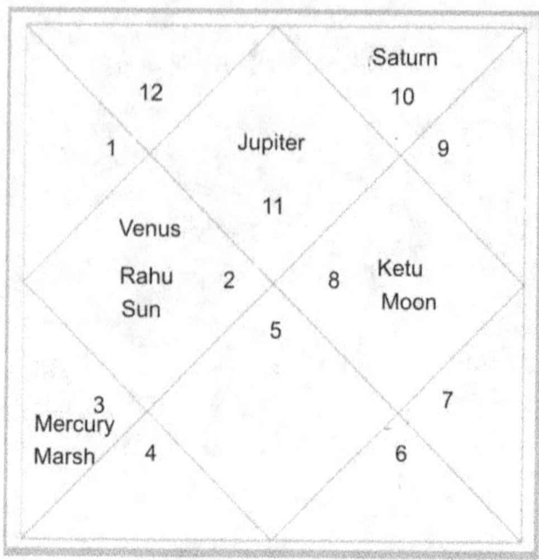

Now Venus will be under the effects of Rahu, ketu and Sun. Mercury will be under the effect of Marsh. Moon will be under the effect of Rahu, Ketu and Sun. however as Jupiter will not be under the effect of any of the rough planet, so Covid-19 cases will go on decreasing.

On 28th May 2021, Venus will move into Gemini zodiac group.

78

<u>**Planetary   position on 28th May 2021 (As per Indian Astrology)----**</u>

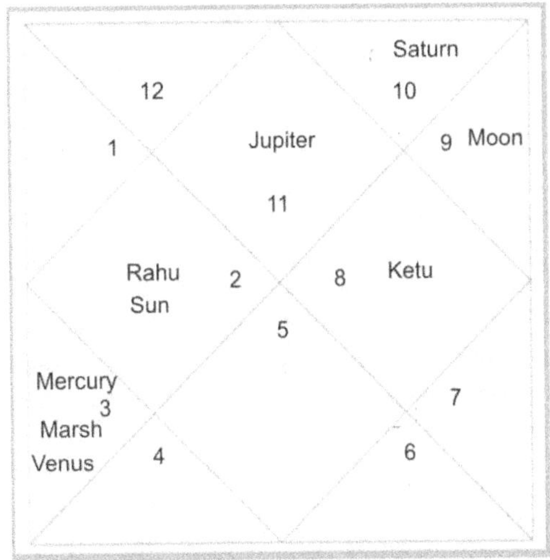

Now Venus and Mercury will be under the effect of Marsh. Full seventh sight of Marsh will be on Moon. But as Jupiter will not be under the effect of any of the rough planet, so Covid -19 cases will go on decreasing.

On 2nd June 2021, Mercury will move into Taurus zodiac group with retarding motion and Marsh into Cancer zodiac group.

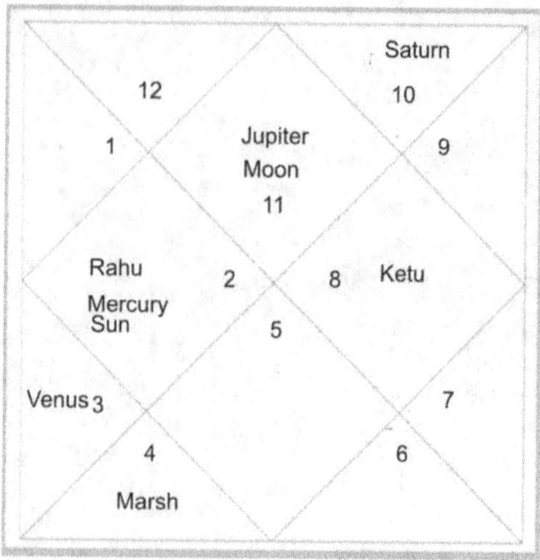

Now full eighth sight of Marsh will be on Jupiter and Moon. Mercury will be under the effects of Rahu, Ketu and Sun. But as Venus will not be under the effect of any of the rough planet, so Covid-19 infection will go on decreasing.

On 16th June 2021, Sun will move into Gemini zodiac group.

<u>**Planetary position on 16th June 2021 (As per Indian Astrology)---**</u>

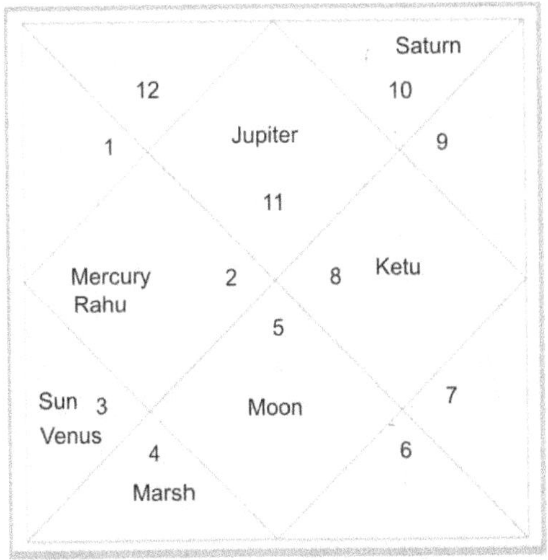

Now Mercury will be under the effects of Rahu and Ketu. Venus will be under the effect of Sun. Full eighth sight of Marsh will also be on Jupiter. As except Moon, all other three soft planets will be under the effects of rough planets, so Covid-19 infection will go on increasing.

On 23rd June 2021, Venus will move into Cancer zodiac group.

81

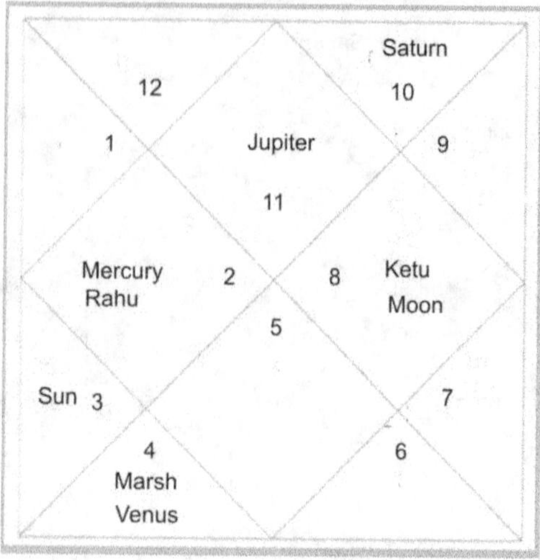

Now Venus will be under the effect of Marsh. Full ninth sight of Ketu will also be on Venus. Mercury will be under the effects of Rahu and Ketu. Moon will be under the effects of Rahu and Ketu. Full eighth sight of Marsh will be on Jupiter. As all the four soft planets are under the effects of rough planets, so Covid-19 cases will go on increasing.

On 7th July, Mercury will move into Gemini zodiac group.

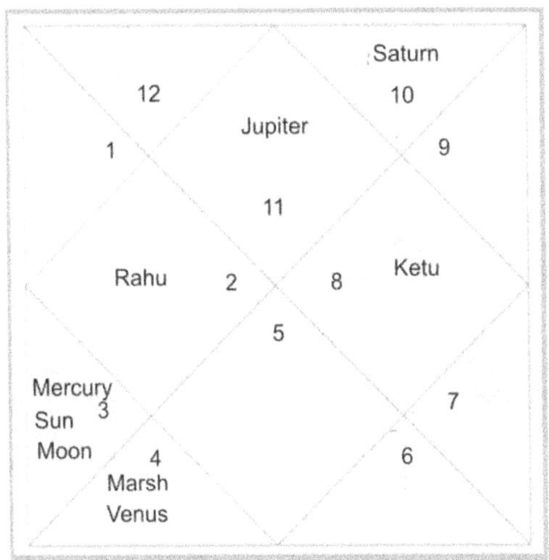

Now Mercury and Moon will be under the effect of Sun. Venus will be under the effect of Marsh. Full ninth sight of Ketu and full seventh sight of Saturn will be on Venus .Full eighth sight of Marsh will be on Jupiter. As again all the four soft planets will be under the effects of rough planets, so Covid-19 cases will go on increasing.

On 17th July 2021, Sun will move into Cancer and Venus into Leo zodiac group.

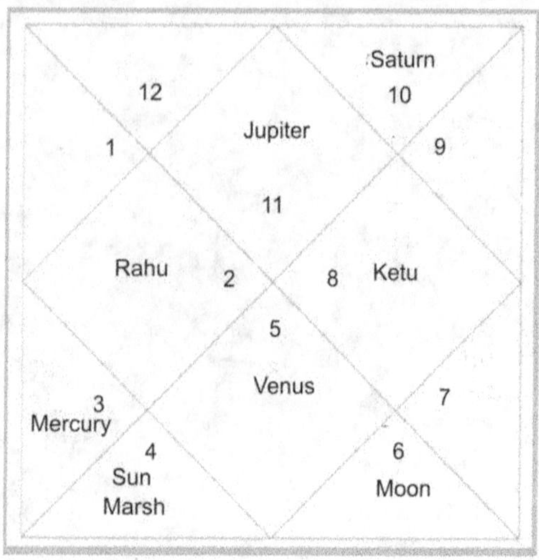

Now full fifth sight of Rahu will be on Moon and full eighth sight of Marsh will be on Jupiter. But as Venus and Mercury will not be under the effect of any of the rough planet, so Covid-19 cases will start decreasing.

On 21st July 2021, Marsh will move into Leo zodiac group.

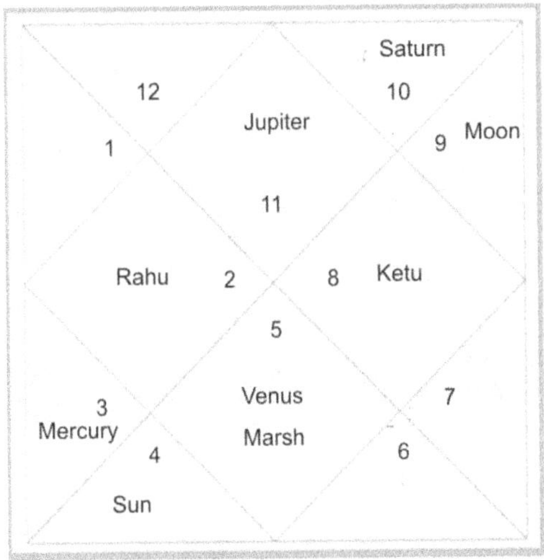

Now full seventh sight of Marsh will be on Jupiter, Venus will be under the effect of Marsh. But as Mercury and Moon will not be under the effect of any rough planet, so Covid-19 infection will go on decreasing.

On 26th July 2021, Mercury will move into Cancer zodiac group.

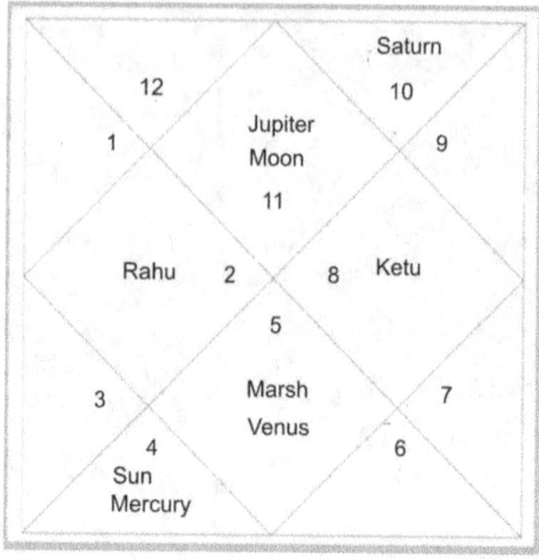

Now full seventh sight of Marsh will be on Jupiter and Moon. Mercury will be under the effect of sun. Full seventh sight of Saturn will also be on Mercury. Venus will be under the effect of Marsh.

As all the four soft planets are under the effect of rough planets, so Covid-19 cases will now go on increasing.

On 9th August 2021, Mercury will move into Leo zodiac group.

Planetary   position on 9th August   2021 (As per Indian Astrology)—

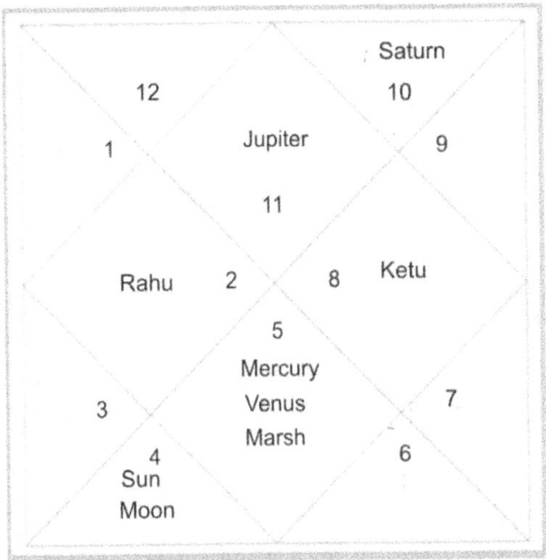

Now full seventh sight of Marsh will be on Jupiter . Moon will be under the effect of Sun. Full ninth sight of Ketu will also be on Moon. Venus and Mercury will be under the effect of Marsh. As all the four soft planets will be under the effects of rough planets, so Covid-19 cases will go on increasing.

On 12th August, Venus will move into Virgo zodiac group.

<u>**Planetary   position on 12th August 2021 (As per Indian Astrology)----**</u>

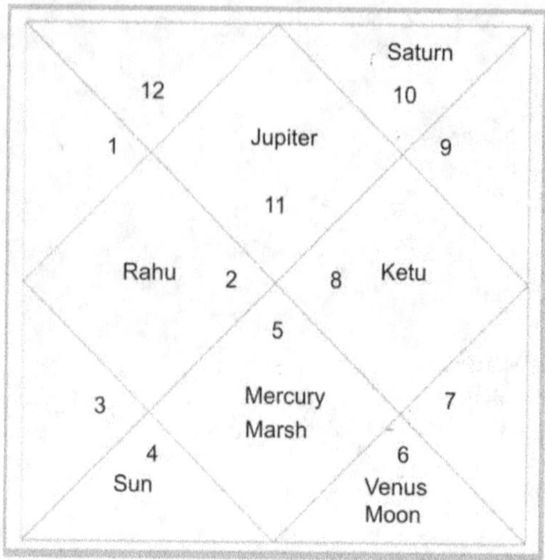

Now full seventh sight of Marsh will be on Jupiter. Mercury will be under the effect of Marsh. Full fifth sight of Rahu will be on Venus and moon. As all the four soft planets will be under the effect of rough planets, so Covid-19 cases will go on increasing.

On 17th August 2021, Sun will move into Leo zodiac group.

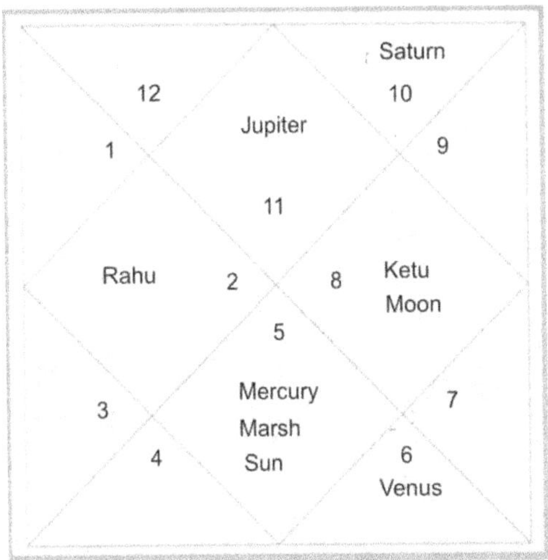

Now full seventh sights of Sun and Marsh will be on Jupiter. Mercury will be under the effects of Sun and Marsh. Full fifth sight of Rahu will be on Venus. Moon will be under the effect of Rahu and Ketu.

As still all the four soft planets will be under the effects of rough planets, so Covid-19 cases will go on increasing.

On 27th August 2021, Mercury will enter into Virgo zodiac group.

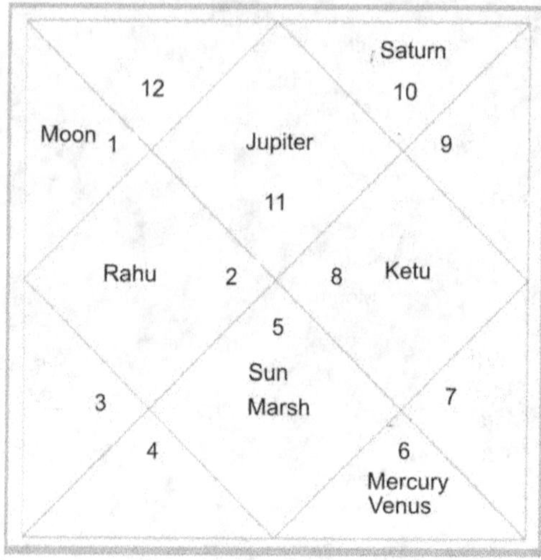

Now full seventh sight of Sun and Marsh will be on Jupiter. Full fifth sight of Rahu will be on Mercury and Venus. Despite Moon will not be under the effect of any of the rough planets, but as other three soft planets will be under the effects of rough planets, so Covid-19 cases will go on increasing.

On 6th Sept. 2021, Marsh will move into Virgo and Venus into Libra zodiac group.

<u>**Planetary position on 6th Sept. 2021 (As per Indian Astrology)----**</u>

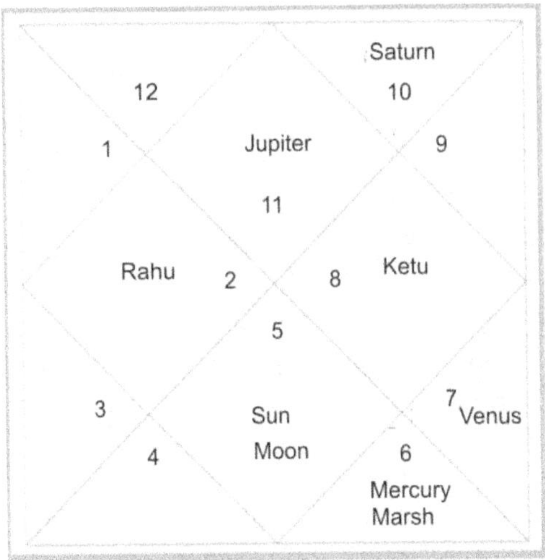

Now Moon will be under the effect of Sun, full seventh sight of Sun will be on Jupiter. Mercury will be under the effect of Marsh, full fifth sight of Rahu will also be on Mercury. Full tenth sight of Saturn will be on Venus.

As all the four soft planets will be under the effects of rough planets, so Covid-19 cases will go on increasing.

On 15th Sept. 2021, Jupiter will move into Capricorns zodiac group with retarding motion.

<u>**Planetary   position on 15th Sept.   2021 (As per Indian Astrology)---**</u>

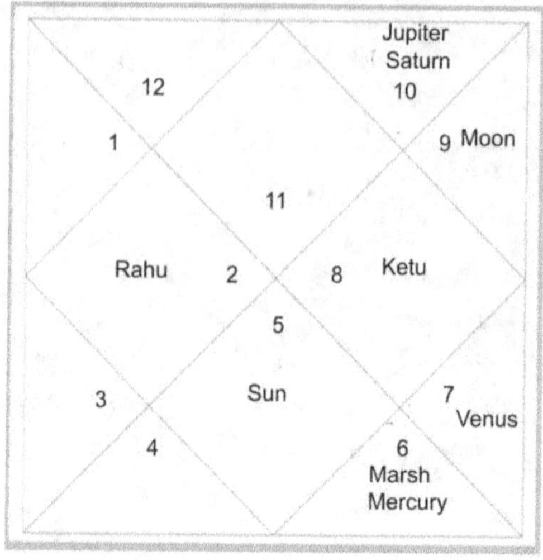

Now Jupiter will be under the effect of Saturn, full ninth sight of Rahu will also be on Jupiter. Full fourth sight of Marsh will be on Moon. Mercury will be under the effect of Marsh, full fifth sight of Rahu will also be on Mercury. Full tenth sight of Saturn will be on Venus.

As all the four soft planets will be under the effects of rough planets, so Covid-19 cases will increase drastically.

On 17th Sept. 2021, Sun will move into Virgo zodiac group.

<u>**Planetary position on 17th Sept. 2021 (As per Indian Astrology)—**</u>

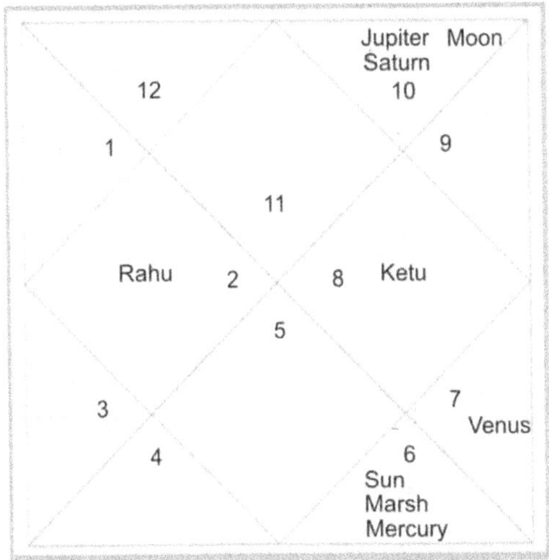

Now Jupiter and Moon will be under the effect of Saturn , ninth full sight of Rahu will also be on Jupiter and Moon. Mercury will be under the effects of Sun and Marsh. Full tenth sight of Saturn will be on Venus. As all the four rough planets are under the effects of rough planets, so Covid-19 cases will go on increasing.

On 22nd Sept. 2021, Mercury will move into Libra zodiac group.

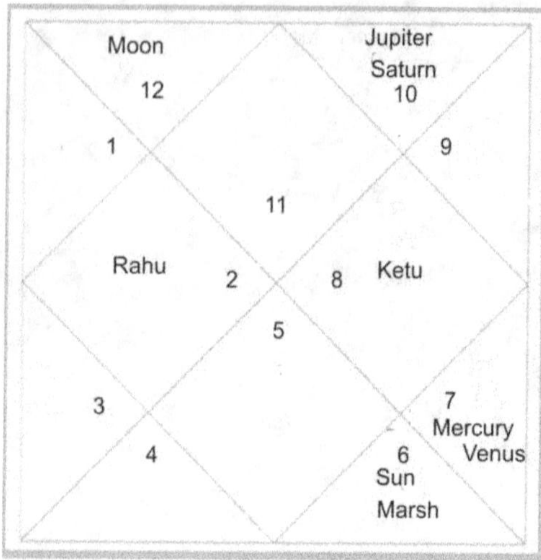

Now Jupiter will be under the effect of Saturn, full ninth sight of Rahu will alo be on Jupiter. Full third sight of Saturn and fifth sight of Ketu will be on Moon. Full tenth sight of Saturn will be on Mercury and Venus.

As still all the four soft planets will be under the effects of rough planets, so Covid-19 cases will go on increasing.

On 2nd Oct. 2021, Mercury will move into Virgo zodiac group with retarding motion and on 3rd Oct. 2021, Venus will move into Scorpio zodiac group.

<u>**Planetary   position on 3rd Oct 2021   (As per Indian Astrology)----**</u>

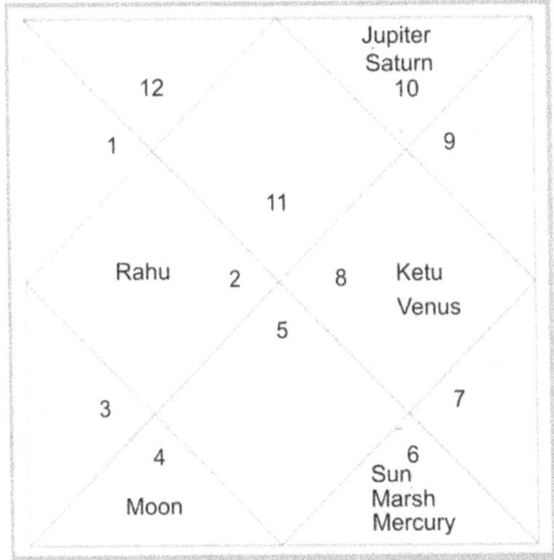

Now full seventh sight of Saturn and ninth sight of Ketu will be on Moon. Mercury will be under the effects of Sun and Marsh, full fifth sight of Rahu will also be on Mercury. Venus will be under the effect of Rahu and Ketu. Jupiter will be under the effect of Saturn and full ninth sight of Rahu will also be on Jupiter.

As all the four soft planets will be under the effects of rough planets, so Covid-19 cases will go on increasing.

On 17th Oct. 2021,Sun will move into Libra zodiac group.

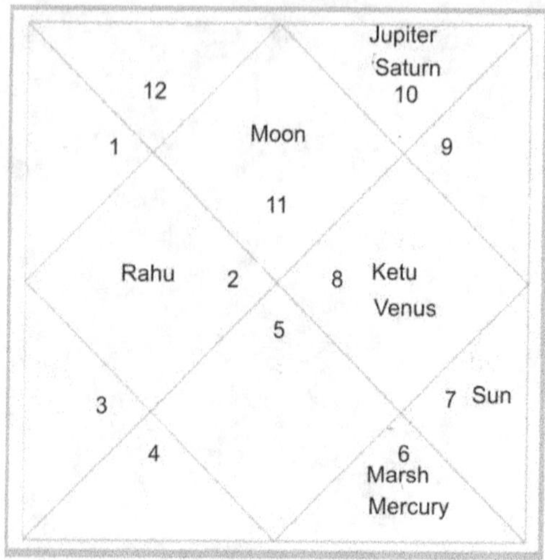

Now Jupiter will be under the effect of Sun, full ninth sight of Rahu will also be on Jupiter. Venus I will be under the effects of Rahu and Ketu. Mercury will be under the effect of Marsh and full fifth sight of Rahu will also be on Mercury. As except Moon all other three soft planets will be under the effects of rough planets, so Covid-19 cases still will go on increasing.

On 22nd Oct. 2021, Marsh will move into Libra zodiac group.

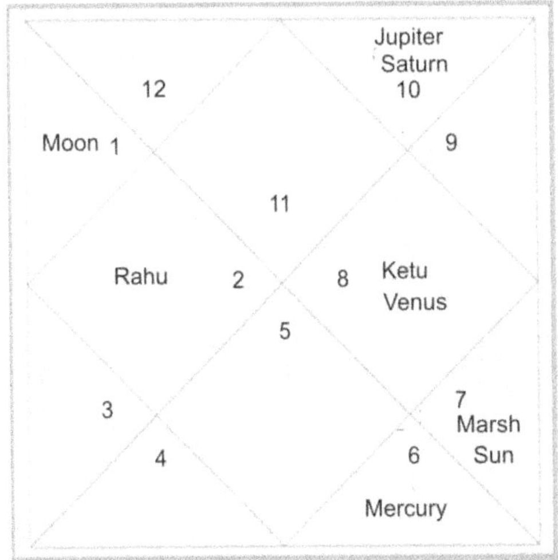

Now, full seventh sights of Sun and Mercury will be on Moon. Jupiter will be under the effect of Saturn, full ninth sight of Rahu and fourth sight of Marsh will also be on Jupiter. Venus will be under the effects of Rahu and Ketu. Full fifth sight of Rahu will be on Mercury. As all the four soft planets will be under the effects of rough planets, so still Covid-19 cases will go on increasing.

On 31st Oct. 2021, Venus will move into Sagittarius zodiac group.

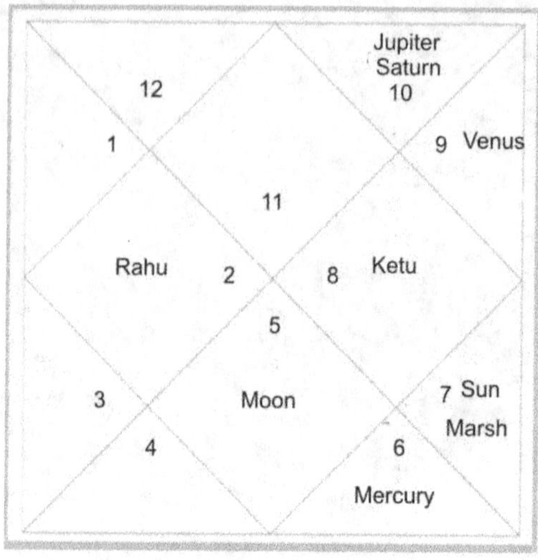

Now Jupiter will be under the effect of Saturn, full ninth sight of Rahu and fourth sight of Marsh will also be on Jupiter. Full fifth sight of Rahu will be on Marsh. However as Moon and Venus will not be under the effect of any of the rough planets, so now Covid-19 cases will start decreasing.

On 3rd Nov. 2021, Mercury will move into Libra zodiac group.

<u>**Planetary position on 3rd Nov. 2021   (As per Indian Astrology)----**</u>

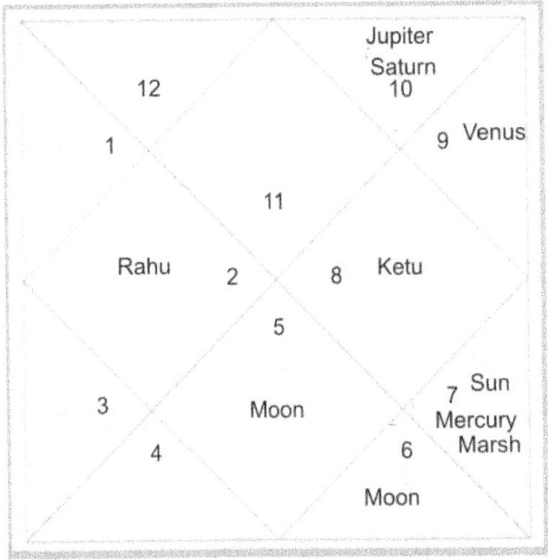

Now fifth sight of Rahu will be on Moon. Mercury will be under the effects of Sun and Marsh, full tenth sight of Saturn will also be on Mercury .Jupiter will be under the effect of Saturn, full ninth sight of Rahu and fourth sight of Marsh will also be on Jupiter. But as soft planet Venus will not be under the effect of any of the rough planets, so Covid-19 case will go on decreasing.

On 17th Nov. 2021, Sun will move into Scorpio zodiac group.

<u>**Planetary position on 17th Nov. 2021   (As per Indian Astrology)-**</u>

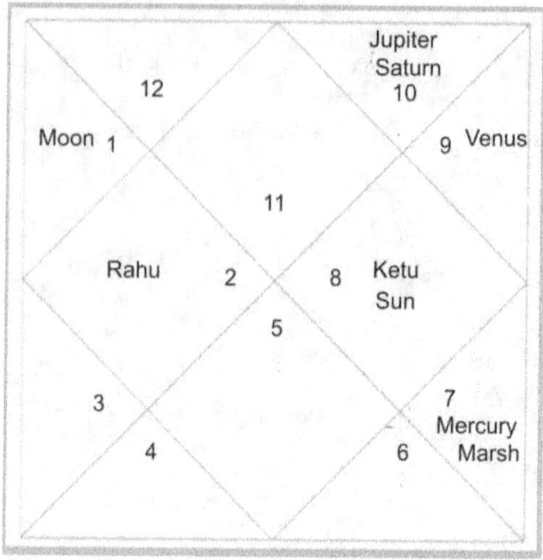

Now full seventh sight of Marsh will be on Moon. Mercury will be under the effect of Marsh, full tenth sight of Saturn will also be on Mercury. Jupiter will be under the effect of Saturn and full ninth sight of Rahu and fourth sight of Marsh will also be on Jupiter. But as Venus will not be under the effect of any of the rough planets, so Covid-19 cases will go on decreasing.

On 21st Nov. 2021, Mercury will move into Scorpio zodiac group.

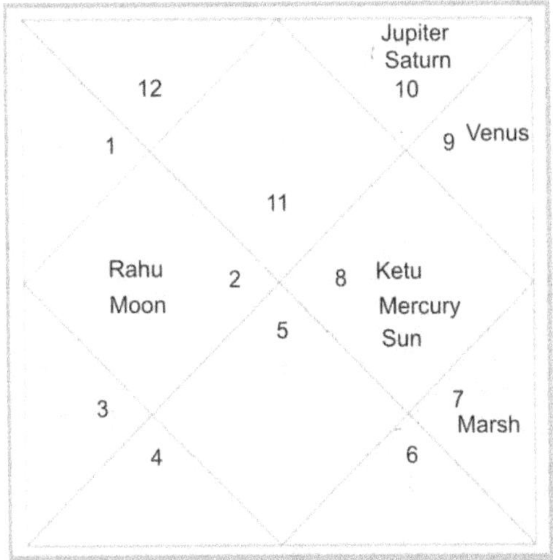

Now Moon will be under the effects of Rahu and Ketu, full seventh sight of Sun and eighth sight of Marsh will also be on Moon. Mercury will be under the effects of Sun, Rahu and Ketu. Jupiter will be under the effect of Saturn, full ninth sight of Rahu and fourth sight of Marsh will also be on Jupiter. But as Venus will not be under the effect of any of the rough planets, so Covid 19 cases will go on decreasing.

On 22nd Nov. 2021, Jupiter will move into Aquarius zodiac group.

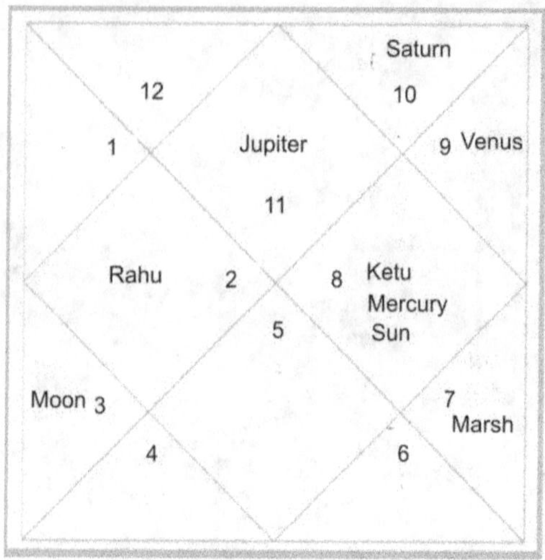

Now Mercury will be under the effects of Sun, Rahu and Ketu .But as soft planets Jupiter, Venus and Moon will not be under the effects of any of the rough planets,so Covid-19 cases will go on decreasing drastically.

On 5th Dec. 2021, Marsh will move into Scorpio zodiac group.

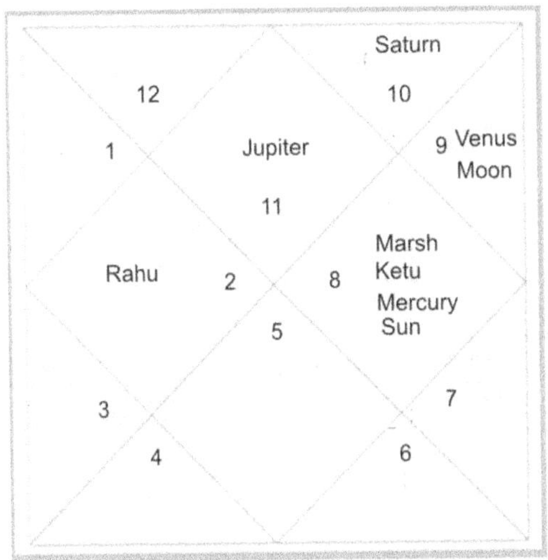

Now full fourth sight of Marsh will be on Jupiter. Mercury will be under the effects of Rahu, Ketu, Sun and Marsh. But as soft planets Venus and Moon will not be under the effect of any of the rough planets, so Covid-19 cases will go on decreasing.

On 9th Dec. 2021, Venus will move into Capricorns zodiac group.

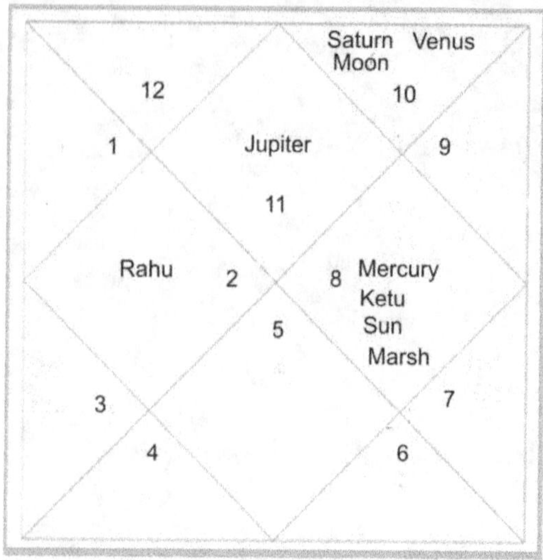

Now full fourth sight of Marsh will be on Jupiter. Venus and Moon will be under the effect of Saturn, full ninth sight of Rahu will also be on Venus and Moon. Mercury will be under the effects of Rahu, Ketu, Sun and Marsh. As all the four soft planets will be under the effects of rough planets, so Covid-19 cases will go on increasing .

On 10th Dec. 2021, Mercury will move into Sagittarius zodiac group.

<u>**Planetary position on 10th Dec. 2021 (As per Indian Astrology)—**</u>

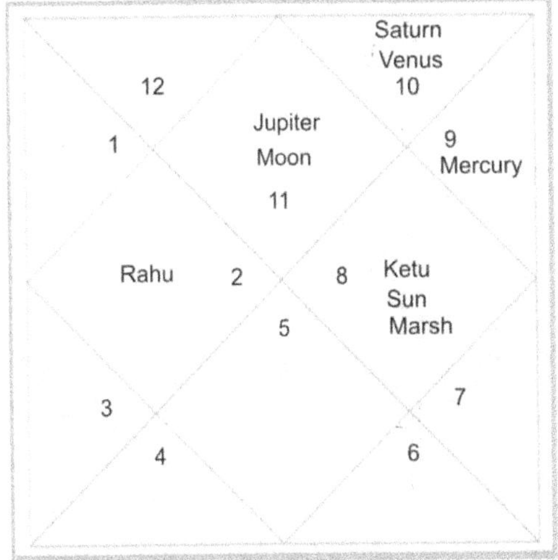

Now full fourth sight of Marsh will be on Jupiter and Moon. Venus will be under the effect of Saturn, full ninth sight of Rahu will also be on Venus. But as Mercury will not be under the effect of any of the rough planets, so again Covid-19 cases will be increasing.

On 17th Dec. 2021, Sun will move into Sagittarius zodiac group.

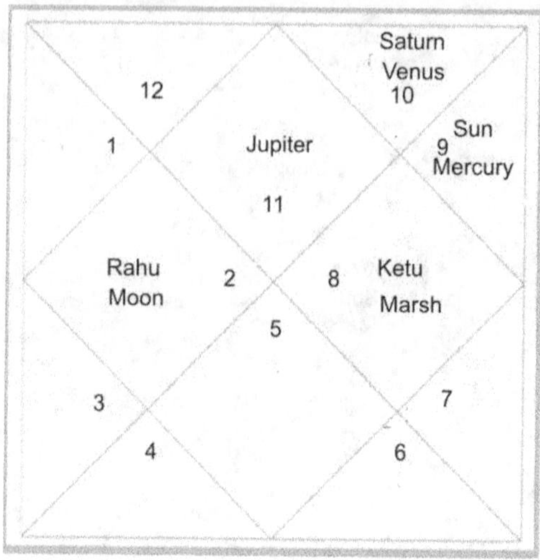

Now full fourth sight of Marsh will be on Jupiter. Moon will be under the effects of Rahu, Ketu , full seventh sight of Marsh will also be on Moon. Mercury will be under the effect of Sun, Venus will be under the effect of Saturn. As all the four soft planets will be under the effects of rough planets, so again Covid-19 cases will be increasing.

On 26th Dec. 2021, Mercury will move into Capricorns zodiac group.

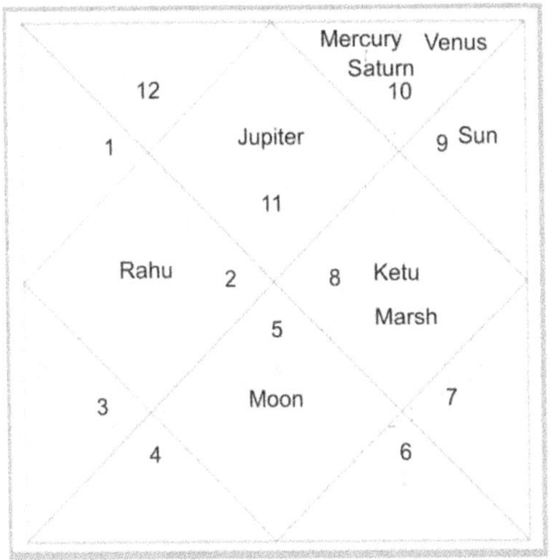

Now full fourth sight of Marsh will be on Jupiter. Venus and Mercury will be under the effect of Saturn, full ninth sight of Rahu will also be on Venus and Mercury. As except Moon, other three planets will be under the effects of rough planets, so Covid-19 cases will go on Increasing.

On 30th Dec. 2021, Venus will move into Sagittarius zodiac group with retarding motion.

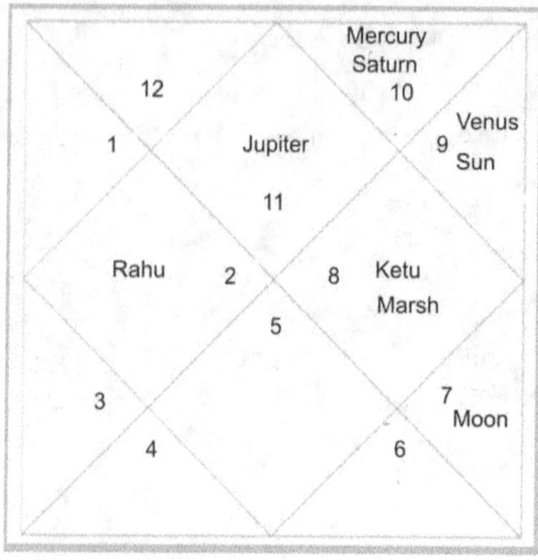

Now full tenth sight of Saturn will be on Moon. Venus will be under the effect of Sun. Mercury will be under the effect of Saturn, full ninth sight of Rahu will also be on Mercury. Full forth sight of Marsh will be on Jupiter. As all the four soft planets will be under the effect of rough planets, so Covid-19 cases will go on increasing.

On 15th Jan. 2022, Sun will move into Capricorns zodiac group.

<u>**Planetary   position on 15th Jan. 2022 (As per Indian Astrology)----**</u>

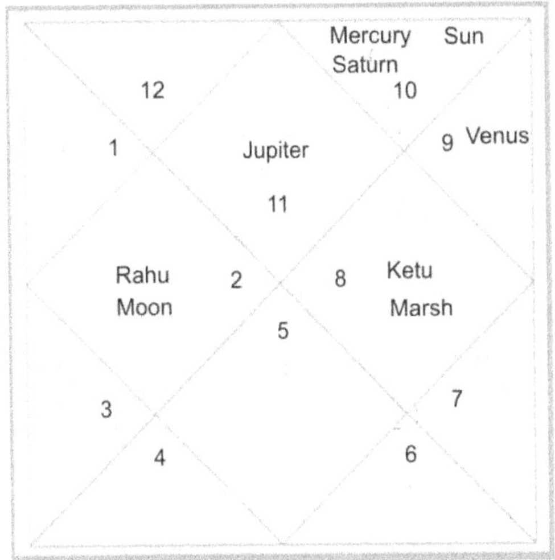

Now Moon will be under the effects of Rahu and Ketu, full seventh sight of Marsh will also be on Moon .Full fourth sight of Marsh will be on Jupiter. Mercury will be under the effects of Sun and Saturn. However as the soft planet Venus will not be under the effect of any of the rough planet , so Covid-19 cases will start decreasing.

On 17th Jan. 2022, Marsh will move into Sagittarius zodiac group.

<u>**Planetary   position on 17th Jan. 2022 (As per Indian Astrology)----**</u>

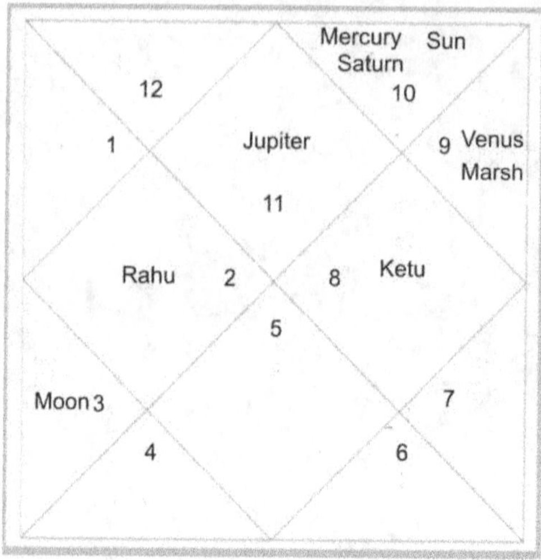

Now full seventh sight of Marsh will be on Moon. Venus will be under the effect of Marsh. Mercury will be under the effects of Saturn and Sun, full ninth sight of Rahu will also be on Mercury. However as the planet Jupiter will not be under the effect of any of the rough planets, so Covid-19 cases will now go on decreasing.

On 13th Feb. 2022, Sun will move into Aquarius zodiac group.

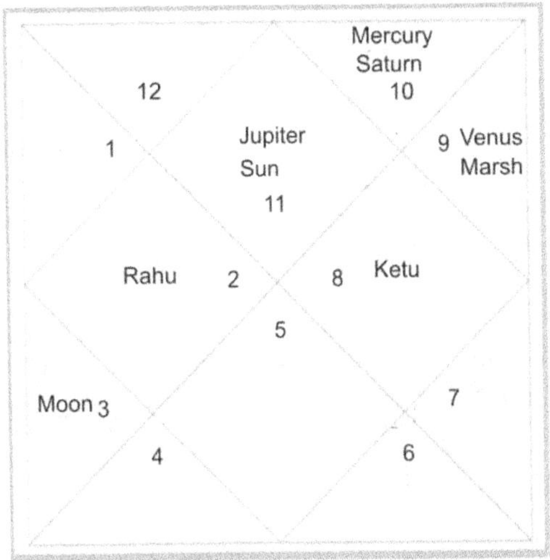

Now full seventh sight of Marsh will be on Moon. Venus will be under the effect of Marsh. Mercury will be under the effect of Saturn, full ninth sight of Rahu will also be on Mercury. Jupiter will be under the effect of Sun. As all the four soft planets will be under the effect of rough planets, so Covid-19 cases will now go on increasing.

On 27th Feb. 2022, Marsh and Venus wil move into Capricorns zodiac group.

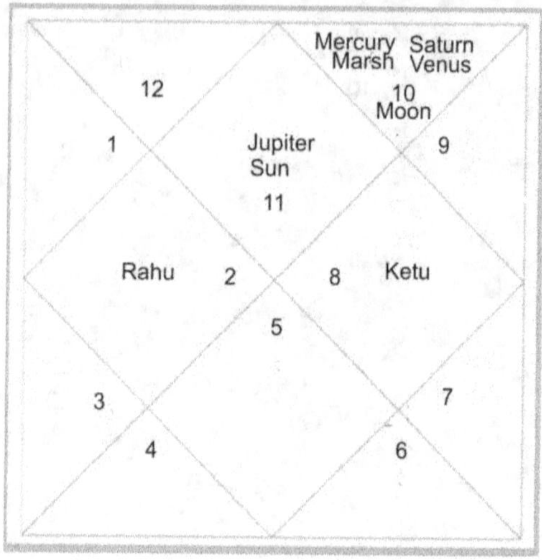

ow Jupiter will be under the effect of Sun. Mercury, Venus and Moon will be under the effect of Saturn and Marsh. Full ninth sight of Rahu will also be on Mercury, Venus and Moon. As all the four soft planets will be under the effect of rough planets, so Covid-19 cases will go on increasing.

On 7th March, 2022, Mercury will move into Aquarius zodiac group.

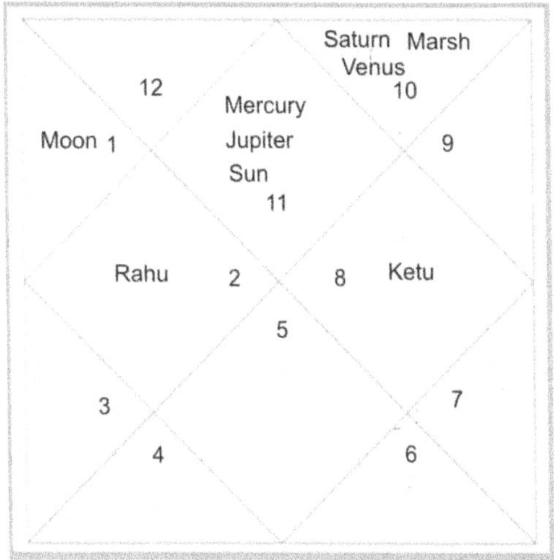

Now Mercury and Jupiter will be under the effect of Sun. Venus will be under the effect of Saturn and Marsh. As except Moon , other three soft planets will be under the effect of rough planets, so Covid-19 cases will still go on increasing.

On 15th March 2022, Sun will move into Pisces zodiac group.

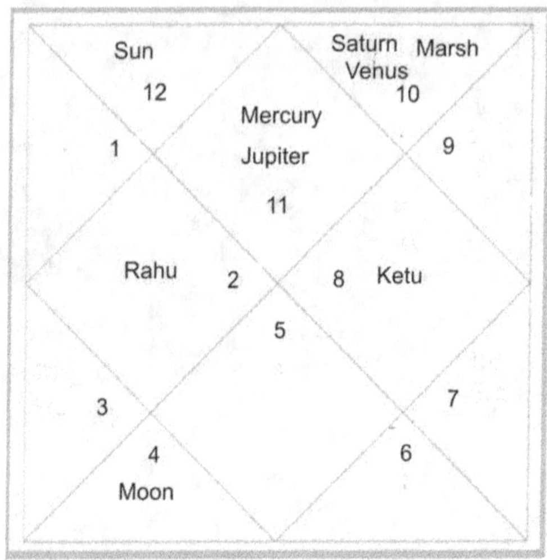

Now full seventh sights of Saturn and Marsh will be on Moon, full ninth sight of Ketu will also be on Moon. Venus will be under the effect of Saturn and Marsh, full ninth sight of Rahu will also be on Venus .But as Jupiter and Mercury will not be under the effect of any of the rough planets, so Covid-19 cases will now be decreasing.

On 24th March 2022, Mercury will move into Pisces zodiac group.

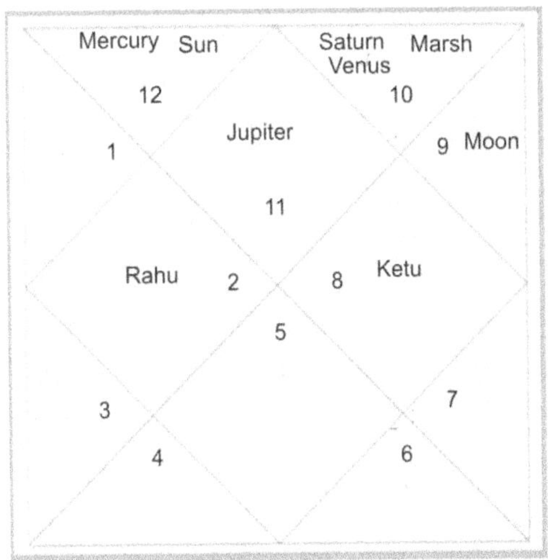

Now Mercury will be under the effect of Sun, full fifth sight of Ketu and full third sight of Saturn will be on Mercury. Venus will be under the effects of Saturn and Marsh, full ninth sight of Rahu will also be on Venus. But as Moon and Jupiter will not be under the effect of any of the rough planets, so Covid-19 cases will go on decreasing.

On 30th March 2022, Venus will move into Aquarius zodiac group.

Planetary position on 30th March 2022 (As per Indian Astrology)----

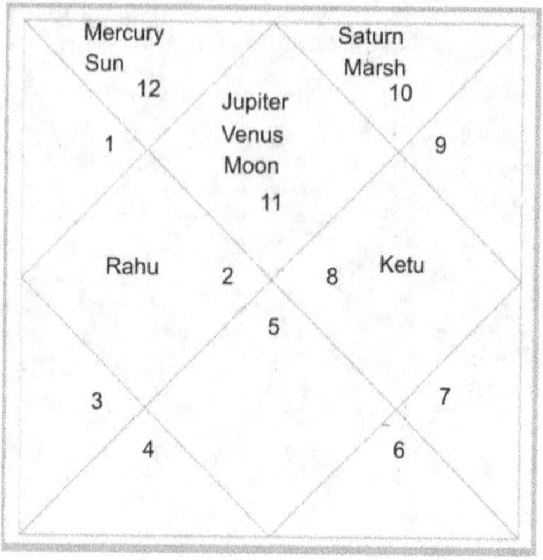
Mercury
Sun
12
Saturn
Marsh
10
Jupiter
Venus
Moon
11
1
9
Rahu
2
8
Ketu
5
3
7
4
6

Now Mercury will be under the effect of Sun, full fifth sight of Ketu and full third sight of Saturn will also be on Mercury. But as soft planets Moon, Venus and Jupiter will not be under the effect of any of the rough planets, so Covid-19 cases will be decreasing drastically.

On 7th April 2022, Marsh will move into Aquarius zodiac group.

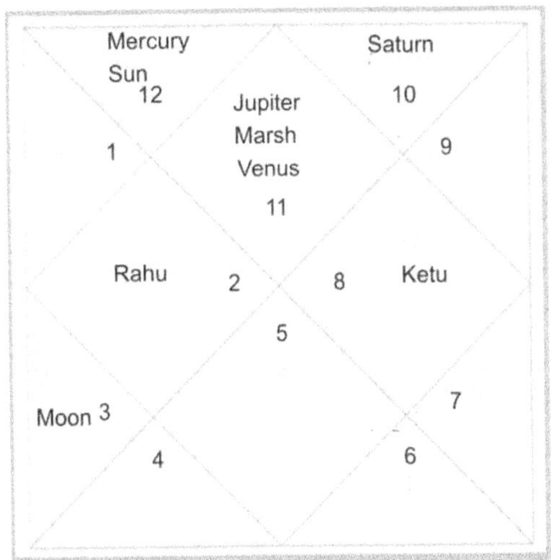

Now Mercury will be under the effect of Sun, full fifth sight of Ketu and third sight of Saturn will also be on Mercury. Jupiter and Venus will be under the effect of Marsh . As except Moon, other three soft planets will be under the effect of rough planets, so Covid-19 cases will start increasing.

On 8th April 2022, Mercury will move into Aries zodiac group.

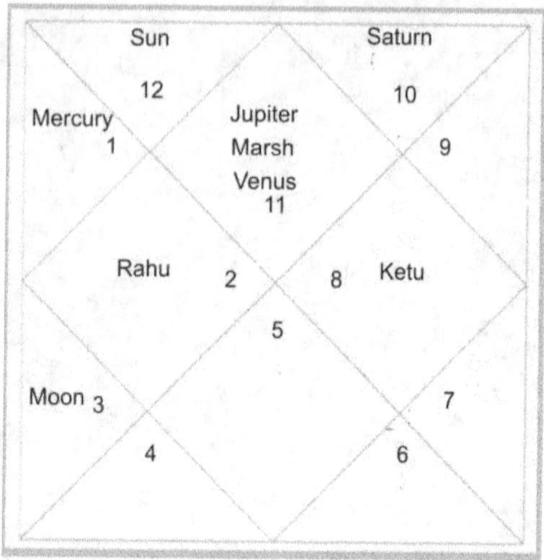

Now Jupiter and Venus will be under the effect of Marsh. As soft planets Mercury and Moon will not be under the effect of any of the rough planets, so Covid-19 cases will start decreasing.

On 11th April 2022, Rahu will move into Aries and Ketu into Libra zodiac groups.

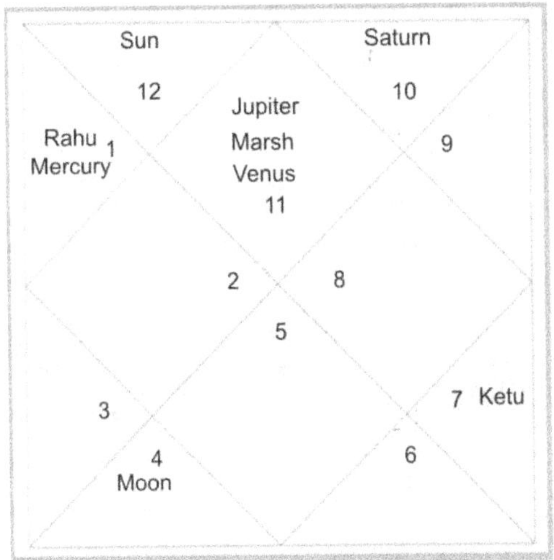

Now full seventh sight of Saturn will be on Moon. Mercury will be under the effect of Rahu and Ketu. Venus and Jupiter will be under the effect of Marsh. Full fifth sight of Ketu will also be on Jupiter and Venus. As all the four soft planets will be under the effects of rough planets, so Covid-19 cases will now go on increasing.

On 13th April 2022, Jupiter will move into Pisces zodiac group.

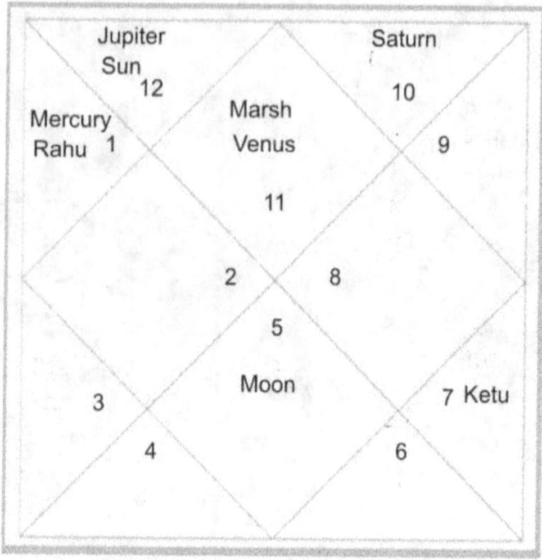

Now Jupiter will be under the effect of Sun, full third sight of Saturn will also be on Jupiter. Venus will be under the effect of Marsh, full fifth sight of Ketu will also be on Venus. Mercury will be under the effect of Rahu and Ketu. Full fifth sight of Rahu and full seventh sight of Marsh will be on Moon. As all the four soft planets will be under the effects of rough planets, so Covid-19 cases will go on increasing drastically.

On 14th April 2022, Sun will move into Aries zodiac group.

<u>**Planetary position on 14th April 2022 (As per Indian Astrology)----**</u>

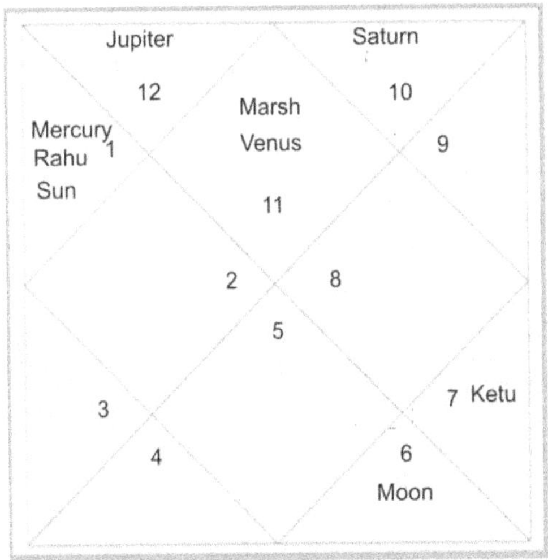

Now Venus will be under the effect of Marsh, full fifth sight of Ketu will also be on Venus. Full third sight of Saturn will be on Jupiter. Mercury will be under the effects of Sun, Rahu and Ketu. Full eighth sight of Marsh will be on Moon. As all the four soft planets will be under the effects of rough planets, so Covid-19 cases will go on increasing drastically

On 24th April 2022, Mercury will move into Taurus zodiac group.

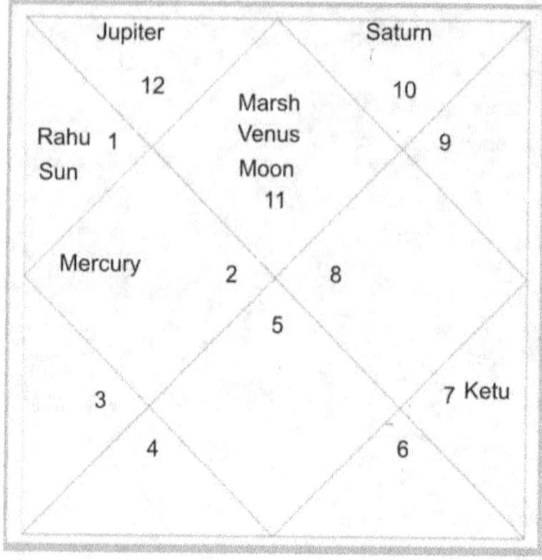

Now full third sight of Saturn will be on Jupiter. Venus and Moon will be under the effect of Marsh, full fifth sight of Ketu will also be on Venus and Moon .Full fourth sight of Marsh will be on Mercury. As all the four planets will be under the effects of rough planets, so Covid-19 cases will go on increasing drastically.

On 27th April 2022, Venus will move into Pisces zodiac group.

<u>**Planetary   position on 27th April   2022 (As per Indian Astrology)---**</u>

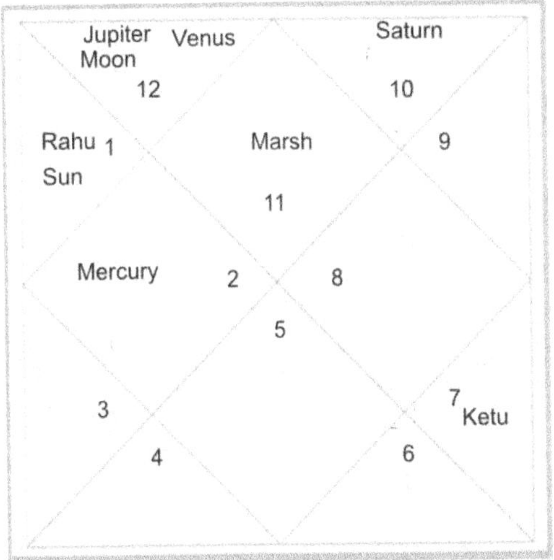

Now full fourth sight of Marsh will be on Mercury. Full third sight of Saturn will be on Jupiter, Venus and Moon. As all the four soft planets will be under the effects of rough planets, so Covid-19 cases will go on increasing.

On 30th April 2022, Saturn will move into Aquarlus zodiac group.

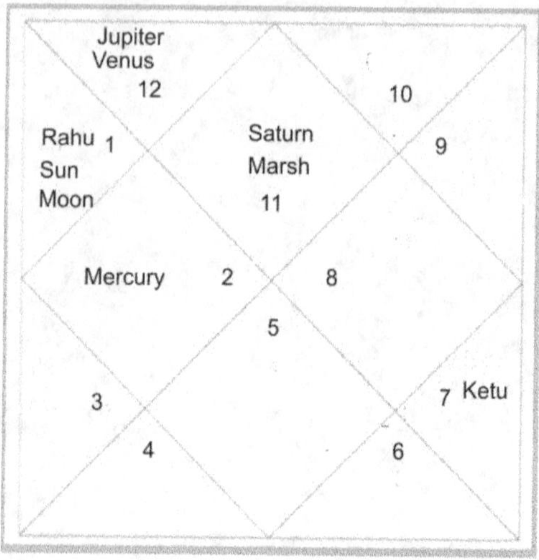

Now full fourth sight of Marsh will be on Mercury, Moon will be under the effects of Rahu, Ketu and Sun. However as soft planets Jupiter and Venus will not be under the effects of any of the rough planets, so now Covid-19 cases will be decreasing drastically.

On 14th May 2022 Sun will move into Taurus zodiac group.

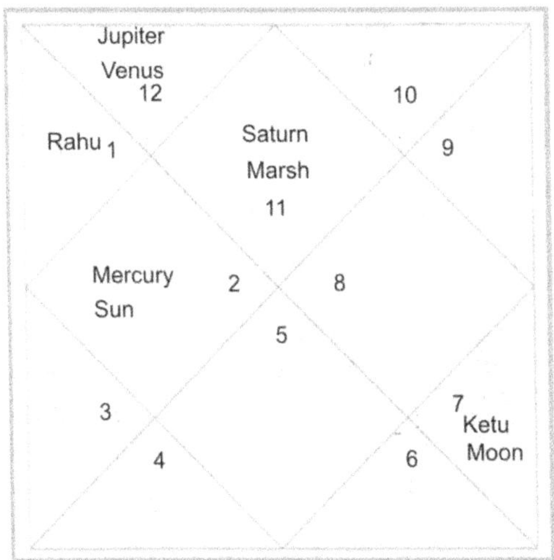

Now Moon will be under the effects of Rahu and Ketu. Mercury will be under the effect of Sun. However as soft planets Jupiter and Venus will not be under the effect of any of the rough planets, so Covid-19 cases will go on decreasing.

On 17th May 2022, Marsh will move into Pisces zodiac group.

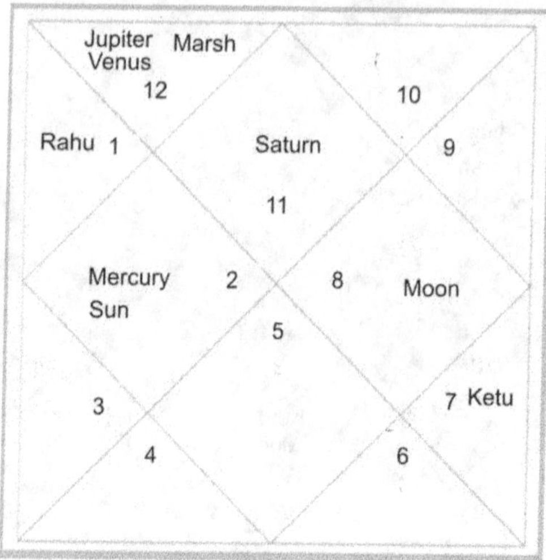

Now full seventh sight of Sun will be on Moon, Mercury will be under the effect of Sun. Jupiter and Venus will be under the effect of Marsh. As again all the four soft planets will be under the effects of rough planets, so again Covid-19 cases will be increasing.

On 23rd May 2022, Venus will move into Aries zodiac group.

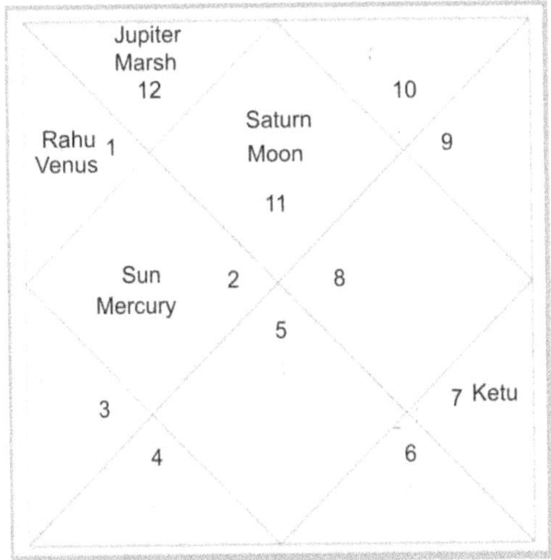

w Moon will be under the effect of Saturn, full fifth sight of Ketu will also be on Moon. Jupiter will be under the effect of Marsh. Venus will be under the effects of Rahu and Ketu, third full sight of Saturn will also be on Venus. Mercury will be under the effect of Sun. As still all the four soft planets will be under the effects of rough planets, so Covid-19 cases will go on increasing.

On 15th June 2022, Sun will move into Gemini zodiac group.

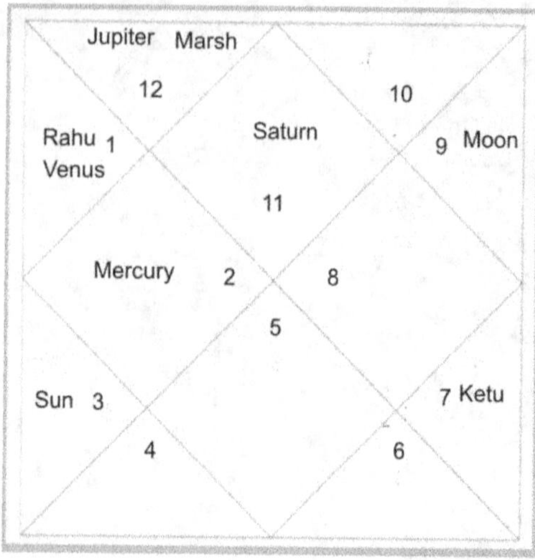

Now full seventh sight of Sun and full ninth sight of Rahu will be on Moon. Jupiter will be under the effect of Marsh. Venus will be under the effects of Rahu and Ketu . However as Mercury will not be under the effect of any of the rough planets, so now Covid-19 cases will start decreasing.

On 18th June 2022, Venus will move into Taurus zodiac group.

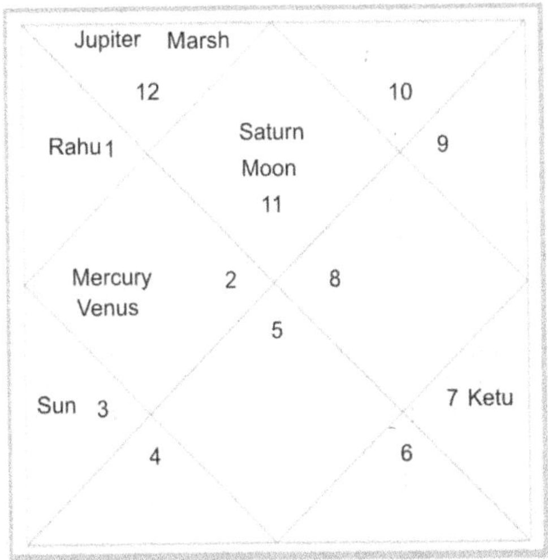

Now Moon will be under the effect of Saturn, full fifth sight of Ketu will also be on Moon. Jupiter will be under the effect of Marsh. But as soft planets Venus and Mercury will not be under the effect of any of the rough planets, so now Covid-19 cases will start decreasing.

On 27th June 2022, Marsh will move Into Arles zodiac group.

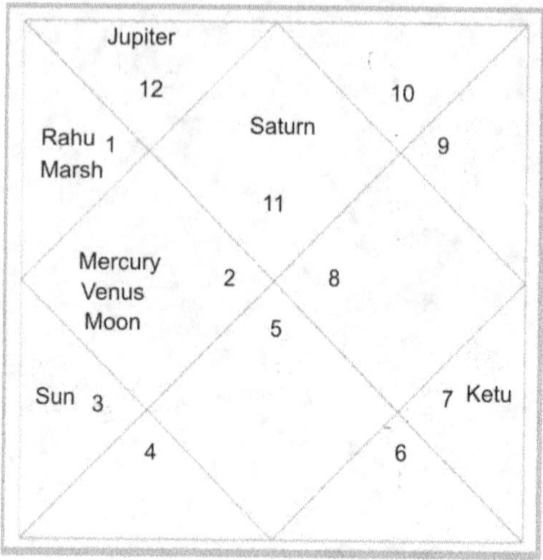

Now as none of the soft planets- Jupiter, Mercury, Venus or Moon will be under the effect of any of the rough planets- Sun, Marsh, Saturn, Rahu or ketu, so chain of effects of rough planets on soft planets will break, and so Covid-19 infection will come to end.

Chapter 4

Summary

Duration	*Infection Status*
11th Jan.2020 to 12th April 2020	Continuing
13th April 2020 to 24th April 2020	Decrease
25th April 2020 to 18th June 2020	Increase
19th June 2020 to 31st July 2020	Decrease
1st August 2020 to 2nd Sept. 2020	Increase
3rd Sept. 2020 to 16th Sept. 2020	Decrease
17th Sept. 2020 to 23rd Sept. 2020	Increase
24th Sept. 2020 to 20th Nov. 2020	Decrease
21st Nov. 2020 to 14th Jan. 2021	Increase
15th Jan. 2021 to 5th Feb. 2021	Decrease
6th Feb. 2021 to 14th March 2021	Increase

Period	Effect
15th March 2021 to 1st April 2021	Decrease
2nd April 2021 to 5th April 2021	Increase
6th April 2021 to 15th June 2021	Decrease
16th June 2021 to 16th July 2021	Increase
17th July 2021 to 25th July 2021	Decrease
26th July 2021 to 30th Oct. 2021	Increase
31st Oct. 2021 to 8th Dec. 2021	Decrease
9th Dec. 2021 to 14th Jan. 2022	Increase
15th Jan. 2022 to 12th Feb. 2022	Decrease
13th Feb. 2022 to 14th March 2022	Increase
15th March 2022 to 6th April 2022	Decrease
7th April 2022	Increase
8th April 2022 to 10th April 2022	Decrease
11th April 2022 to 29th April 2022	Increase
30th April 2022 to 16th May 2022	Decrease
17th May 2022 to 14th June 2022	Increase
15th June 2022 to 26th June 2022	Decrease
27th June 2022	End of Corona (Covid-19) virus Effect

Biblography

The author is a "Graduate Electronics Engineer" (B.Tech.) from Birla Institute of Technology, Mesra, Ranchi, India. The author has more than 25 years of experience as an amateur astrologer. The author has developed many new concepts in Indian Vedic astrology. The author has interest in writing atrological articles on earthquakes, landslides, cyclones, weather , political and wars predictions.

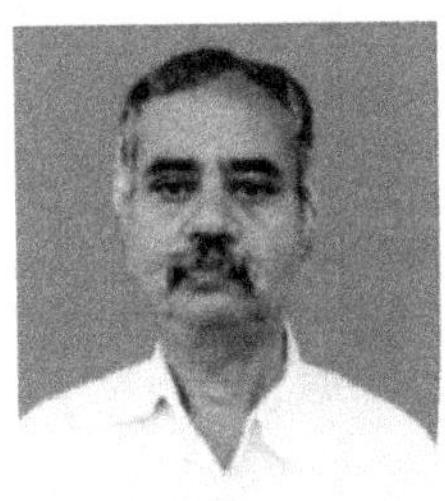

PS

www.ingramcontent.com/pod-product-compliance
Lightning Source LLC
Chambersburg PA
CBHW060105260726
48658CB00004B/1408